ALL MY SINS REMEMBERED

and

THE OTHER SIDE OF GENIUS

ALL MY SINS REMEMBERED
Another Part of a Life

and

THE OTHER SIDE OF GENIUS
Family Letters

WILFRED R. BION

EDITED
BY
FRANCESCA BION

Routledge
Taylor & Francis Group
LONDON AND NEW YORK

First published by Fleetwood Prees, 1985
Published 1991 Karnac Books Ltd.

Published 2019 by Routledge
2 Park Square, Milton Park, Abingdon, Oxon OX14 4RN
52 Vanderbilt Avenue, New York, NY 10017

First issued in hardback 2019

Routledge is an imprint of the Taylor & Francis Group, an informa business

ISBN 13: 978-0-367-10700-0 (hbk)
ISBN 13: 978-1-85575-845-2 (pbk)

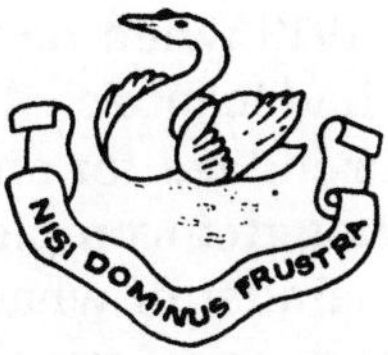

Bion family crest
Nisi dominus frustra

'Except the Lord build the house, they labour in vain that build it: except the Lord keep the city, the watchman waketh but in vain.'

Psalm 127. i

FOREWORD

The first volume of Wilfred Bion's autobiography, *The Long Week-end*, covered the period up to 1919 when he was demobilized from the army and for the first time had to face civilian life as an adult, unqualified for any profession, or indeed for any occupation by which he might earn his living. Although incomplete and only in first draft, I wanted to publish the remainder of what he wrote; but it leaves us with a thirty-year blank and, even more unfortunately, an abiding impression of unrelieved gloom and profound dislike of himself.

This sad, self-searching testimony would on its own present a false picture of the life of a man who came to derive great happiness and reward from his marriage, family and work. The clearest evidence of this is provided by his letters to us, written with no audience in mind and no need to lay stress on his sins of omission, confident of our love and understanding. Almost all his creative thinking and writing were done during these years when he was at last released from the confines of war, bereavement and a sense of hopelessness.

We make public some of these private communications because they tell the reader so much—not about us, his wife and children, but about him, the husband and father. We are proud to have been his family and the recipients of his love.

Francesca Bion
Abingdon, Oxfordshire.
1984

FOREWORD TO *THE LONG WEEK-END*

Wilfred Bion was born in Muttra, in the United provinces of India, in 1897. Many generations of his family (of Huguenot descent) had served in India—as missionaries, in the Indian Police, and in the Department of Public Works. At the age of eight he was sent to England to attend preparatory school, never again to return to India. All his life he retained a strong affection for the country of his birth; he died in November 1979 two months before a planned visit to Bombay.

His autobiography was left unfinished, but the years covered by this book form a distinct period which ended with demobilization just before he went up to Oxford to read History. He felt then that he had to start life again, building on unsure foundations. He regarded himself as uneducated, out of touch with the world outside school and the army, and demoralized by his experience of war. Nevertheless his outstanding athletic ability in rugger and swimming saved the day—just as it had done during his schooldays.

Although he felt that the war had left him unable to take advantage of the opportunities offered at the university, he always recalled with gratitude the talks he had with H. J. Paton, the philosopher. By 1924 it was clear to him where his interests lay—in psycho-analysis. He started medical training at University College Hospital, London, won the Gold Medal for Surgery, qualified in 1930, and then went on to psycho-analytic training. At University College Hospital he had contact with another outstanding man, Wilfred Trotter, the surgeon and author of *Instincts of the Herd in Peace and War*. Both Paton and Trotter played a very great part in his intellectual development.

After the Second World War, during which he served as the Senior Psychiatrist on the War Office Selection Board, he devoted the rest of his life to the practice of psycho-analysis. He became one of the foremost original thinkers in this field, and also in that of group behaviour, lecturing widely and writing prolifically—many papers and some fourteen books, most of which are now required reading in training institutes.

He was Chairman of the Executive Committee of the Tavistock Clinic, London, in 1945; Director of the London Clinic of

Psycho-analysis from 1956-62; and President of the British Psycho-analytical Society from 1962-65.

In 1968 a request that he work in Los Angeles provided the opportunity to escape from what he called 'the cosy domesticity' of England. The vast open spaces of the western United States awoke in him memories of his childhood in India: the culture, however, was altogether new to him. It released him from the confines of traditionalism and enabled him to entertain his 'wild thoughts'; his mind was as wide open to new impressions during the last decade of his life as it had ever been in youth. So it was that in the alien, vital, dangerous but superficially idyllic environment of California he was stimulated to write the trilogy, *A Memoir of the Future,* a psycho-analytically oriented autobiographical fantasy—the most controversial and least understood of his works.

The qualities of courage and leadership, already evident by the time he was twenty years old, stood him in good stead as a psycho-analyst. He made plenty of enemies, as original thinkers always do, but no amount of hostility ever deflected him from his determination to be true to himself and to his beliefs.

Although he originally intended to stay only three or four years in California, he did not return to England until 1979. He died two months later in Oxford, with the 'dreaming spires' visible from his hospital bed.

Those who were fortunate enough to be touched by his wisdom and affectionate concern were never quite the same again. We who knew him well will carry something of him with us for the rest of our lives.

Francesca Bion
Abingdon, Oxfordshire.
1982

ALL MY SINS REMEMBERED

Another Part of a Life

1

OXFORD University, at which I found myself the next day—my mother having already returned to India by the earliest boat on which she could find a passage—was a prospect that had aroused feelings of awe since the day I had been granted an exhibition; so the reality of Oxford railway station came as a shock. A hundred or so undergraduates milled around looking for their luggage. Once it would have been porters they sought, but now there were no porters and no wealthy golden youth to employ them. In army style we went directly to the barrows, the trunks, and hopefully to the taxi queue.

Thus opened for me a period of unparalleled opportunities to which I remained obstinately blind. I was overwhelmed before I started by the aura of intellectual brilliance with which Oxford was surrounded. Actual contact with my contemporaries intensified my sense of inadequacy. They came from schools with famous names; I did not. They came from homes with a university tradition; I did not. "Here comes Bion with his non-conformist hat on", was the kindly jest with which a fellow in my rugger team greeted my arrival to board the bus for an 'away' match. It embarrassed me, but it also brought some relief—at least it was not that bloody 'college cap'. No one said, "You there, you wearing that pious mug on your face, na poo! Finish! 'op it!" Oxford was very kind and tolerant.

"Oh, by the way," one distinguished interviewer had said, coming to the end of his time and, I suspect, his resources for believing in my suitability as a candidate, "any intitials?" I was puzzled. I thought hard. At last light dawned.

"Oh, W. R."

It was his turn to be puzzled. "W.R.?.No, no! I mean MC or something."

Feeling extremely embarrassed, I owned up to the DSO and ultimately the Legion of Honour. I explained that the latter was almost unavoidable as I had been in action "near the French"—as if I had contracted something contagious or infectious. He looked at me incredulously, glanced at his notes on my record—which was athletically outstanding if nothing else—and decided at last that it made sense. Obviously Dumb. I think we were both relieved. After I had escaped from the room I wondered if *he* had the Legion of Honour. It was only too likely.

My lack of brains, or I suppose I should call it 'intelligence', now began to be a serious source of anxiety. I remembered how much it had worried me at school although I had maintained a degree of painful anonymity because of my great skill at games and by my being placed, probably through despair of finding any suitable niche for me, in what was called the Sixth Form (History Specialists). These—there happened to be only one and I was 'it'—were understood to be scholarship candidates for one of the two main universities.

The army had given me a short respite from the shame and fear of sex, though there too I feared death in action would come to me as a sign of God's wrath and final requital. Now the whole ghastly business was back again. Games, thank God, again to the rescue. DSO, Mention in Dispatches, Legion of Honour—all very fast-fading reassurances, which at best had failed dismally to convince me, although they had a wistfully reassuring effect on those who contemplated my heroic qualities as manifested in their effulgence. Blown up, I assumed heroic proportions concealing a scholar, concealing an athlete, concealing a physical wreck, the fast diminishing victim of 'self-abuse' concealing 'masturbation', 'expulsion' and, most terrifying of all, 'General Paralysis of the Insane'. This last had a certain horrific grandeur about it like Paradise Lost. More often it had no grandeur: like two Canadian undergraduates, baseball enthusiasts, utterly alien objects foreign to everything I understood by the name 'Oxford', who had as their theme song an endlessly reiterated tuneless ditty, 'Ashes to ashes, and dust to dust; if the wine don't get you then ... the women must.'

How we laughed! Those were the days! How shocked they were in the bar of that little pub! All except one fellow. Ah, but he was a knowing one. He was the manager of a small travelling theatrical company. He became confidential one evening in the Common Room and told the two Canadians, his hosts, that they could have any one of the pretty girls in the choruses he engaged, or else ...! He made an expressive gesture; "Oh, they know all right. Believe me they know what it is to find themselves without a job—these days!" The small fat Canadian began to drool; the tall one's eyes became hard. I was a hardened prig, but not so hard as to stop the anxiety mounting uncontrollably as I wondered why I felt so ignorant, so shocked. 'Dominus illuminatio mea'; my eyes travelled down to Oxford's towers.

Oxford was wonderful. Some power must reside in that 'Dominus illuminatio mea'—like 'Quo fata vocant, quo fas et gloria ducunt'—which could never be overwhelmed, not even by the unspeakable misery that seemed always to be threatening. There was nothing heroic about that misery; just utter loneliness and menace, the more frightening because there was nothing there, nothing more comprehensible than the snigger of a sexual joke. The theatrical manager reminded me of Clifford, the same knowing narrowed eyes, the would-be smart suit, the pointed cheap shoes and, I suspected, the same buoyant personality with a supply of self-esteem ready to flow into and instantly seal up any puncture which might lead to deflation. There were no other such visitors to our Junior Common Room.

One day in the High I saw a familiar figure, small, dapper, well-cut hacking jacket, finely polished boots, a disdainful sneer. I called out his name before I could stop myself. I knew he had seen me, but clearly had not heard me. For so small a man it was wonderful that he could command so great a height from which to look down upon Oxford and its dwarfs. "They have gone", I could almost hear his mournful bleat "Even my dear friend the Prince." But he had some wit; at least, I thought his Tank Corps Marching Song was amusing:

We'll all go a-tanking today,
For fruits of their marriage we'll pray.
If it's not a Rolls Royce
Which I'd pick out for choice,
Then a nice little Ford bright and gay.

I'm sorry he cut me dead; at the time I felt I might have helped restore his wounds, for at least I preferred him to the far bulkier, heavier mass of bounderdom that had threatened to horsewhip him. In fact I could have done nothing for that terrible depth of misery and isolation. Where do butterflies go when the climate becomes inclement?

The poor Major. I see him now, dapper in the sunlight as he turned away from this figure from his past. But I was not as disreputable as he thought, and not as disreputable and shoddy as I was to feel when again I was to suffer rejection—far more serious than anything he could inflict upon me even in his days of glory as Adjutant.

I met Quainton in Oxford one day; he was attending a Workers' Education Conference. It did not occur to me to ask if he ever met the Major, though since they admired each other they might have established a continuing friendship, and the fact that both were sheepishly superior to me might have been compatible with a curious similarity in the lack of common interest that I felt. It was not a repulsion—that suggests something too positive—but a cold glazing of the eyes as if a thin film separated us and prevented what might have become a mutual hatred.

"How are things?" I asked Quainton awkwardly.

"Oh, fine", he replied. "Fine", he repeated with a lack-lustre insincerity.

We did not meet again. How well I remembered my envy of his frank open ways, his charm, his privileged position with the Major. "Fine!" "How are things?" "Oh fine!" The words form the epitaph for a friendship which promises fair but turns sour and ends in disillusion.

I went into the Parks. It was a lovely day; sunny, with a few fine weather clouds glowing in the blue sky. I had some time to spend for I was early for a meeting with a friend with whom I was going swimming. As I lay on the grass and waited, my mind wandered to the bleak cold and darkness of Ypres and how grateful I had felt to Quainton for his cheerfulness and sturdiness at that dark time. What a change had come: I wished I could help him as some small way of being grateful. It was impossible to get past those lustreless eyes; to talk more after that "Fine!" was an intrusion when one had been warned, "Keep off!"

Carter had come to see me a week or two before. I liked him and he liked me. He and Hauser and I had, unlike Quainton, lasted the war. *That* barrier did not exist, yet barrier there was. We could not reminisce about the war; and we had nothing else to talk about. Hauser and I never met again and we did not correspond. I could not imagine that we would write or meet even if the opportunity had come. It seemed impossible that our shared war could mean so little: yet that appeared to be the case. But I soon realized it was not so: the experience, however short the meeting, was not forgotten; I could forget names but I could not forget the people.

2

NEWMAN was in his study—the same that had once been the Holy of Holies of poor God-Almighty Shaw. He welcomed me and very soon we were talking about his House and its affairs. I thought he was ill at ease. His wife came in and we had tea. She was a large, florid woman, unattractive by virtue of a prominent robust Roman nose—rather like a bird of prey I thought. Her brother was the music master who had been one of the heroes of myself in common with my contemporaries and previous generations of school fellows, the composer of the militant Christian battle hymn of 'Onward Christian So-ho-ho-hol-jers on to the cookhouse door!' He and Newman were great friends and so it was no surprise that a romance had sprung up between Newman and the musician's sister. It was said, in keeping with Newman's well-known loyal and statistical bent, that he boasted that their union bound together four school families and their seventeen genealogues.

It was not an easy party. I was awed by weight of reminiscent but somehow jaded grandeur. It was not simply that the lady's beauty was of a kind that eluded me, clothed as it was in the fleshy armour of rectitude, but ... but ... well, when she had gone and tea had been cleared away, Newman leant forward and in confidence laid bare the mystery: he had taken to drink. In shocked and almost whispered terms he confessed. I suppressed an impulse to laughter, which was so out of keeping with his unmistakably serious distress. I had noticed that he had offered me a glass of sherry before lunch; he had I think even taken one himself. I remembered thinking at the time, how unlike the school I had known before the war when the puritan sanctity could not have been invaded by—sh—alcohol. Alas; Oxford and the West Front had disguised from my own eyes the deterioration in my moral standards, a deterioration so great that I had not even observed the depravity of my old friend—for even as a schoolboy I had been very fond of him. I thought he looked and was as nice and amusing as ever.

Later his brother-in-law gradually made matters clear. His sister, whom he felt fraternally obliged to protect, led an awful life though she never betrayed it behind her front of cheerful calm. Of course he, partly to preserve the innocence of his old pupil, could not tell me but hinted at terrible things which were masked behind the divinity of poor old Newman—'Dr' Newman. He blew his nose, but inadvertantly in pulling out his handkerchief he had dropped a condom on the floor—he was wearing his dressing-gown preparatory to going to bed. Smartly he slid a slippered foot over the offending object lest my insatiable curiosity should be prompted into activity. I had learned years before from Misses Evans and Cuff to keep a glaze handy for slipping over my tell-tale eyes. I did *not* see—well, not much you know—not really, if you see what I mean—y'know.

Nevertheless, I did not see; I did not see that peacetime was no time for me. I did know, however many pretty ribbons I put on a wartime uniform, that wartime also was no time for me. I was twenty-four; no good for war, no good for peace, and too old to change. It was truly terrifying. Sometimes it burst out in sleep. Terrified. What about? Nothing, nothing. Oh well, yes. I had a dream. I dug my nails into the steep and slippery walls of mud that fell sheer into the waters of a raging, foaming Steenbeck. Ridiculous! That dirty little trickle? If blood is thicker than water, what price the thickness of dreams? Suppose broad daylight was not thick enough to keep out the terror. Suppose I was so terrified that I ran away when it was really a battle. I woke up. Was I going crazy? Perhaps I *was* crazy.

There was a boy in the school whom I liked. He was intelligent, a fair athlete and used sometimes to have tea with me. I thought he must have a very attractive mother—perhaps a sister. He told me that his mother was coming to visit him; I suggested he should bring her to tea when she came. When the day arrived he said she would be pleased to come. In due course she arrived, alone.

She was a large, gaunt, flushed woman. I thought perhaps she was menopausal. She was shifty, uncommunicative, breathed deeply. I thought she was hostile—didn't like me.

Still, the tea went off all right though she was not the beauty I had hoped for. In fact not very much more beautiful than Newman's consort. Poor Newman—what a battle-axe of a woman. Yet a battle-axe, I reflected, was quite a useful thing to have around if you knew how to wield it, and if the times were not propitious. Not that *I* wanted one.

It was not till the next day that I discovered that times were *not* propitious: the Headmaster wanted to see me in his study. Once I would have trembled at this inauspicious invitation; not now however. I went cheerfully.

He looked grim. He said he had very serious complaints of my behaviour. He had been informed that I had made sexual approaches—Good God! What was this?—to this same boy. Who on earth had said this? The boy, said the Headmaster, when questioned by his mother, had said he "never wanted to see that blighter Bion again."

"But", I said, "she came to tea with me yesterday and I had sent the invitation through him!"

"Yes, well I don't think she should have gone to tea with you, but I want your resignation—I think you should leave the school at once."

I felt my senses had left me. But not all. "No", I said, "I shall be glad to leave at the end of term, but I shall *not* go now."

The interview ended. He would think about it. So would I—if I knew *what* to think about. The time when, filled with panic, we had all run down to the prep school when the gate to the playing field broke? When I had 'run away' and abandoned my tank at Sequehart? The cold and exciting draught at the end of school chapel sermon about poison in a boy's food?

It is true I had had enough of schoolmastering. I would have liked to have had the guts to chuck it up. But to get the sack? No. And certainly not for this nameless crime. One of this Headmaster's favourite questions to a suspect was, "Have you ever grasped his privates?" He had not asked me that, and I remembered how funny—and also repellant—the query seemed to me; I could hardly believe that the story was true. No: I would *not* resign.

Next day the Headmaster told me that since the mother did not want the boy questioned, he could not insist on my immediate removal; I was to leave at the end of the term.

It was a hideous term at a hateful place and I did not know to whom to turn. I realized years later that I should have demanded legal advice in considering the possiblility of an action for damages. But the stormy seas of sex I could not navigate any better than Palinurus. I visited the bottom of this monstrous world beyond the stormy Hebrides. How deceptively calm that term, how friendly were my friends!

It ended, but had I been unfortunate enough to be as wise before the event as after, I might still be the extremely inept and wretched schoolteacher I was then. Who is wise enough to do better than fate?

At the end of that term I went to stay with a friend and on arriving at his home I was met by the most beautiful girl I had ever seen—his sister. She had just finished her last term at school. So had I, but I was not nineteen but twenty-six. I might excusably have been regarded as a mature man of experience and a war hero to boot. She was intelligent and, as I say, beautiful: I was immature and inexperienced except for a passion for a girl at my sister's school. She had been a year older than I, and I was then fourteen. Since then—nothing. My hand trembled when the holiday came to an end and I said goodbye.

"It's awful you must go", she said.

"Perfectly priceless", I blurted out.

"What?" she replied astonished.

I nodded speechlessly to her dress which she had worn particularly for me. Her dismay turned to a joyful laugh.

Later there came a box of wild roses, freshly gathered. Then she came to London to study massage. We met. Irresponsible to the end, I proposed and was accepted; she could not be expected to see through all the war-hero trapping. I could hardly discard the blessed gift of licensed bravery covering the nakedness of which the culture, the mental universe of which I was a part, seemed luckily unaware.

3

"WHY do you want to be a doctor?" the Dean of the medical school inquired. I was not going to say, "Because I want to be a psychoanalyst."

Bertie took his feet off the desk preparatory to telling me there was no vacancy for me as a medical student. In my desperation a voice prompted me to mention I had played rugger for Oxford University. Bertie put his feet back on the desk; we had not finished yet.

"But", I added in a spasm of conscience, "I had to forfeit my Blue because I tore a cartilege in my knee just before the Varsity Match."

Before he had time to take his feet off the desk again, I blurted out that I had captained the Oxford University swimming team. I did not know that the hospital had a swimming team, but I saw that Bertie was again wondering if the unprepossessing mass of ineptitude before him concealed some possibility that had not so far emerged. So did I, though even less hopefully than Bertie. The gold and enamel of the DSO, the bright red ribbon of the Chevalier, did not thaw the freezing cold within. However... in or out? 'In' it was.

But first I had to pass the preliminary examinations in University College, London—the Inter. B.Sc., a trivial exam for any ordinary schoolboy. However, thanks to Oxford University, I had begun to learn that I was uneducated. 'Ob, sub, super, post and pre', said Kennedy's Latin Grammar. 'A right-angled triangle' had various 'properties'. French partitive articles likewise; and ... and ... what else? University College taught me that there *was* nothing else. Back to school I went to learn what I ought to have, but had not, learned.

If I tried to assess my assets I could hardly contemplate the truth; I still wonder how I remained afloat instead of being submerged by my ignorance. I was reputed, wrongly, to be brave—only just having escaped being branded with a cross, bronze, for valour; wooden, to mark the spot where my body lay. I was ignorant alike of love of man or woman. Visibly I was in good health; even mentally I was sombre but not depressed. I did not regard my acceptance by the medical school with any enthusiasm; I cannot now understand the solidity of the foundation of self-satisfaction and complacency that carried me through a period of failure and a prospect of even worse to come. I remained dangerously unaware of the universe in which I continued to live.

When the dons at Oxford spoke of my poor showing in Schools as due to the strain of recent fighting, I assumed that they were trying to be kind about a blockhead. I had a marvellous time, but I did not realize that that was because Oxford was a marvellous university where I had the chance of meeting and forming friendships with people of an age and outlook which could change me for ever. At school Ruskin's *Sesame and Lilies* had opened my eyes to Milton; to those two I have never ceased to have feelings of love and gratitude which no uncomprehending sneers of T. S. Elliot for Milton, nor my inability to grasp Ruskin's *Unto This Last*, nor hints that he was less than perfect, have ever undone.

I had left the army with eyes firmly closed against the possibility that there might be something, known to Milton and Ruskin, beyond the shabbiness of the Great. University College, London (which, it was said, could at most contribute £11 as contrasted with the Queen's College's £260 to undergraduate education) made me feel at home. I did not like its long echoing corridors; I did not like Jeremy Bentham or what he said about his and my old college. Nevertheless I felt that here in this part of London I was more nearly in my class.

I owed much of this to Elliot-Smith who lectured with consummate ease and mastery on the brain. Why I should obtain comfort from that I do not know, for I was fully aware that I could never see my subject so clearly that I could draw a section of the brain as if seen, say, through the sagittal plane, or any other that he chose to illustrate his point. My appreciation of his lectures was the more odd as I did not feel I would ever be able to pass an anatomy exam.

I owed still more to the kindness and generosity of Sir Jack Drummond. He invited me to dinner at his home; he also took me to a dinner at the Savage Club. It was a fascinating evening: the wit and skill of the speakers there was far superior to anything I had heard in my Oxford days. Thanks to Drummond I began to break away from the misery of my athletic failure, my scholastic incapacity, my military inadequacy from which I had been unable to free myself, being tied to it as much by my need to deny it as by lack of any chance to prove otherwise.

There was an unprententious dining club to which Drummond also asked me. The charge for the meal was, I think, three shillings and sixpence and it relied on the College kitchen to provide it. This must have put a strain on the staff, for the kitchen was not usually intended to provide any food beyond lunch for the students, and afternoon tea which was the last meal of the day. On one memorable occasion I was flanked on my left side by Polunin who was then working with Diaghilev's productions of Russian ballet, and on my right by Sir Ronald Ross.

"Diaghilev is a remarkable artist", said Polunin. "I remember when we had completed our rehearsals for the first performance of *Petrouchka*, Stravinsky—who secretly considered the music perfectly able to stand by itself as a work of art and regarded the ballet and decor as redundant—was satisfied. Fokine, who was responsible for the choreography, was similarly pleased. Only Diaghilev was disquieted. 'No', he said, 'it's not quite right.' 'Not right?' said Stravinsky, who was echoed by Fokine. 'Why? What's the matter with it?' they challenged him. Diaghilev said nothing but remained troubled and anxious. Then his expression cleared. 'I've got it! Instead of ending with the death of Petrouchka, his ghost must appear.' The other two went off and considered the matter: Stravinsky to write the extra bars of music; Fokine to arrange that Petrouchka's head and shoulders should appear above the wall waving his drooping arms in final convulsions. They did a last and emended rehearsal and all agreed that Diaghilev was right. That was what made him such a wonderful producer; he could see what the rest of us, absorbed in details, could not see."

Many years later I remembered this story when I saw Carl Ebert's production of Stravinsky's *The Rake's Progress* at Glyndebourne. I wondered if the epilogue to the emotionally searing end, the Rake's death in lunacy, had indeed been unconsciously a consequence of what Stravinsky had learnt from Diaghilev.

It was on this same occasion that Polunin was saying, "I don't expect anyone here would recognize the language of my childhood", when Ronald Ross overheard him and immediately took up the challenge. "Speak a few phrases", he said, and interrupted after the first few words—"Moscow dialect." "Correct", conceded Polunin, who had not met Ronald Ross before.

I was aware that my experience was restorative, but I was not aware of the hurt that needed to be restored; nor of the poison that kept the hurt festering. Today I still do not know; but the conjecture has a quality which distinguishes it from other more benign speculations: the request for my resignation from my old school and, as I later realized, my cowardice in agreeing; the sense of guilt; the bitter resentment at my experience of entertaining to tea a woman who was accepting my hospitality after she had demanded my resignation in a conversation with the Headmaster—the only common feature was sexual dread, which now, with eighty years of experience, I regard as indistinguishable from dreadful sex. For a time it was merely an athletic activity, a muscular movement which made life bearable. In this it contrasted with guilt which made life unpleasurable and did nothing to show me the way to behave unguiltily, unwickedly, unnaughtily.

'The First Class Honours degree for which his tutors hoped was probably impossible after the recent strain of fighting.' What strain? I did not remember any strain—only the disastrous injury to my knee before the Varsity match. Then the shocking disgrace.

But . . . but sir, she has just been to tea with me!

I agree—she shouldn't have done that. But *you* shouldn't have given him an expensive leather pocket book. That was most indiscreet.

But sir, I didn't give him one; all I ever gave was a small notebook with tear-off leaves.

But she said he told her he never wanted to see "that blighter Bion" again.

Had nobody ever come across an adolescent boy who expressed impatience when being badgered by a persistent mother about a schoolmaster of whom he knew nothing and cared less?

What I know now suggests that there is no shortage of people ready to display the many and deplorable qualities of one's physical and mental self. Therefore to swell the number even by one is to make a redundant contribution to what is in any case an uninteresting exhibition. So—why write an autobiography? Because it is interesting to me to review the life I have led in the universe in which I have lived. Just now, for example, I remarked to Francesca—whom I have not yet had reason to mention—on the noise that a small distant plane was making and how sad that on this year's visit to France there seemed to be more than usual of these tiresome gnat-like mechanisms; and she reminded me that when I was staying with Dudley Hamilton in Southend I was as excited as I could very well be because on the last day of my stay we saw a real aeroplane flying! Bleriot had just flown the channel in 1906—some four years before. Four years later it was still exciting to read Belloc's prestigious pronouncements in *Land and Water*. How knowledgeable he was. But not so knowledgeable as Kitchener of course, who made the profound invitation to join the Army for—'Three years *or* the Duration of the War'. It must have been the most intelligent pronouncement that fiercely moustached mouth had ever uttered.

Studying medicine was hard work. I knew what it felt like to be me and to have the feelings that I had, but I had no means of communicating them to a person not myself. I also knew what people not myself looked like; I could only see that they did not appear to be experiencing pain. I learnt what various parts of a cadaver were called. I learnt it 'by heart'. Not so when I saw a girl medical student with shapely legs spread her thighs apart below the level of the dissecting table. *That* observation was not painfully made and I did not have to articulate it. It only required a nudge for my male partner immediately to grasp what I meant. He had no difficulty in appearing to be absorbed in his anatomical study while transferring his gaze from the cadaver to the living thighs. *Cunningham's Anatomy* taught me, with pain and difficulty, to learn what a woman was; my intimidating conscience would not allow me to learn, or even to allow attractive young women to teach me. Who would guess that an ex-soldier (successful), ex-schoolmaster (unsuccessful) did not know what a woman was, and did not know how to find out—except under the discipline of *Cunningham's Anatomy*, and then only in so far as I could exclude the medium of pleasure? I had had the best English Public School education—or so my parents thought. The conclusion would appear, logically, to be inescapable. There must be something wrong with me.

But—the spring wild roses! Of course I knew what they meant—any fool would know that, and what I knew was what any fool would know and not a scrap more. It was at least a year later that an intelligent and wise girl medical student told me with hurt surprise, "I don't think you know what a woman is." She was quite right, and I still had many years of painful learning ahead of me.

I knew that I did not know, but that was a piece of self-knowledge of which I was ashamed and did my best to disprove. When I was chosen to play for the Tank Corps XV at rugger against the French Army team, we had leave for the match including a night in Paris. Our hosts naturally thought that the English He-men would want to go to the Folies Bergères, and as English He-men we were anxious to behave in a manner fitting He-men. I watched, unthrilled, a negro cracking a whip as he drove a supposed team of white women round the stage. Not even an erection—as I feared. One of the professional women came and sat, to my embarrassment, on my knee with her thickly painted face close to my mouth. After a moment or two she began to mock my lack of enterprise. "Ah—trop jeune", she said, not unkindly—my round baby-face needed more than a DSO and Legion of Honour to appear that of a warrior. "Ah, trop jeune", and to my intense relief she got off my knee.

I escaped. But Oxford had no curriculum that would fill the gaps in my essential needs; Oxford had not taught me how basically stupid I was. The donor of the wild roses escaped; it was long before I understood that a girl could be lucky *not* to have married me.

For many years I do not believe I thought of marriage at all. Of what is now recognized as 'sex' I thought a great deal, but it was inseparable from ideas of temptation (nice feelings), madness, purity and high ideals. Having no contact of any kind with girls was easy—I thought they were a mean selection of selfish bitches mostly anxious to tell tales and get brothers into trouble—and contact with boys was restricted to those of unexceptionable morals and preferably athletically successful. However, there were the roses. At the time they were inseparable from 'romance', innocence and love. Later I thought of them, and similarly provocative behaviour, as something that did not cost the donor much. Though it had been painful for me to contemplate any action which cost me thought, consideration and trouble—such as would be involved in finding a box, packing the flowers, taking them to a post office and buying stamps—I did not feel that this involved any such expense of spirit for the girl.

4

OXFORD, London, University College Hospital, Suburbia as usual. I had not realized, and nor had my contemporaries, that the world, the small part of it that was the British Empire, was not as usual, any more than a familiar landscape is 'as usual' just before a Krakatoa erupts. The earth's crust, or the molten sea of lava beneath—as usual?

Just as molton rock solidifies into lava so did the emotional turbulence—white hot energy, revolt, rebellion—cool and solidify into further layers of crystallized debris as it welled up, not only in the world of men and women but also in that minute particle of it of which I have experience and which I am able to observe for myself. As I become aware of thoughts and feelings of my own they become identified. A gross example is this writing which is inseparable from making marks on paper: some of them are marks of a kind which conform to accepted rules of grammar, articulate speech; others do not. I cannot know what it is my intention to record until I have recorded it; and then I shall not know what I have recorded nor what it is of which I am a record. In this respect I do not differ from the fossil which is, unknowingly, the record of something which a sentient being observes and then tries to understand the meaning of what he has observed. So I have, snail-like, left my trace on this piece of paper. If I were a great artist I might leave a sculpture of the god Hermes; it would cause someone to say, "Praxiteles passed this way."

All this is damnably uninteresting. What happened to the girl who sent the roses? Do for God's sake get on with the story.

I am—blast you—if you wouldn't keep interrupting.

I am silent.

What happened to the girl? I wrote to her—I do not now know what. She came to London to study a branch of para-medical skill. I thought I was in love. I proposed marriage one evening inside St James's Park.

It sounds just like Gilbert and Sullivan—'I heard the minx remark she'll meet him after dark and give him one.'[1]

[1] *Iolanthe.*

I thought you were not going to interrupt. Perhaps your comic opera pair would like to take over?

Sorry—do go on.

It was not funny: it hurt. It still does. I had no money, no prospects. No wonder her family didn't want it. They thought she was fooling—just trying out her skills. But her mother said that this time they felt she really meant it. I agreed, but in fact I so little believed it and knew so little about being in love that I did not understand what her mother had said or what the girl meant either by the roses or by "yes". Indeed I had forgotten till now that her mother had been evidence of the genuine sincerity of the girl's response to my proposal.

Well, get on. What next?

It was awful. I had no money; she had no money. She was not qualified; nor was I. I could not learn anatomy or physiology. I felt completely unworthy of the confidence which Sir Jack Drummond had in me; my athletic achievements were a fraudulent passport to being accepted by the Dean of the Medical School. She said good-bye, vowing eternal fidelity, at Victoria Station. What's so funny about that?

I thought Waterloo was your waterloo—excuse the joke.

No, you damned fool—Waterloo was where I left for France after my investiture with the DSO. I had said good-bye to my chalk-complexioned mother an hour before. This was when 'All troops recalled from leave'—when 'our troops were holding the enemy fast in our' (non-existent) 'battle positions'.

I suppose you would have built the Maginot Line?

That war had not even started when I said good-bye at Victoria station.

Go on: I'm thrilled to bits. She vowed eternal fidelity.

Well, no; not exactly. In fact a week or two later I was shocked to have a letter saying she wanted to break off the engagement.

In short, you mean her love had died?

No, you are mixing it up with Betty—and it was not her love that had died. *She* had died. And again I felt I had killed her by not staying with her when her pregnancy was nearing term.

You blamed others for posting you abroad when they could and should have sent some younger analyst?

I did, but they were not to blame. They knew nothing about looking after people over whom they had authority. One of them was going through a crisis in which he was afraid he would not get knighted for his services; another had his time fully occupied in admiring his reflection in the mirror—the Colonel's uniform *is* very seductive.

You seemed to think that about the colonel of your tank battalion before he was reduced to the rank of captain. But what about your *reflection in the mirror in which you saw yourself saying good-bye to Betty?*

At the time I thought she was being very brave although she looked deadly pale. And I reassured her that the West Front, with the war nearly over, was much safer than London or even Bournemouth. The long distance call from Brussels to the War Office brought the reply, "Can you hear me? The baby's very feeble. Can you hear me?"

"Yes, yes"—get on with it blast you; I'm not deaf.

"Betty *died* last Wednesday."

"Thank you very much. No, no, not at all. I can arrange."

You sound very efficient.

I did: I was. Brussels is a nice little town. Betty would like it I am sure. Betty? Dead, he said. She shall not grow old as we who are left grow old. Old; so old. But not improved.

I suppose—although I had the reputation of being somewhat solemn, not to say dull, gloomy and a bit stupid—I have always retained a belief that 'it can't happen to me'. A box where sweets compacted lie.[1] My music shows there is always a 'close' and all must die. But what of it? Death is a characteristic feature of life. And if death is the ultimate fact then logically it is absurd to behave as if it could be avoided. In this respect death is not a matter of practical consequence to anyone, but it is the animate, continuing-to-live object that has to bury or otherwise dispose of the dead object. If your eye offends you pluck it out: if your cancer offends you cut it out: if your mind makes you uncomfortable . . . what then? 'La réponse est le malheur de la question.'[2] So if you have a questioning mind give it an overdose of answers. 'I know', 'Yes, I know': when any of these labels are on the bottle be careful about the dose; learn your psychopharmacy and what truths are lethal.

The girl made sure that I should find out that she had said, "Even from the first I felt my engagement to Wilfred was a mistake; even while I was engaged I felt I was in love with Pat." The dose of venom made it certain that the wound would not be, like a skilful surgical operation, aseptically carried out, but would fester and remain open.

[1] 'Virtue', George Herbert.

[2] Maurice Blanchot.

5

ALFRISTON is a charming village to visit. Lord Amulree invited me to spend a week-end at an abandoned coastguard station, National Trust property, on the cliffs a mile or so to the south-west of Alfriston. At the pub called The Tiger I heard a yokel say, "Yes, my boy's regiment has been posted abroad. Some place they call the Khyber." He hadn't heard of it, but I had; the name Khyber Pass was as familiar to my ears as were the words 'Gordon Highlanders' or 'Kitchener' or the 'Relief March to Khartoum'. Historical debris, like the 'Ridge' on which was our old house in Delhi years after it had been the home of the British Army quelling the 'Mutiny', and of General Dyer who 'saved India by a timely order to fire' at Amritsar. Of course some Indians got killed, but India was 'saved'. My parents found it most disturbing when their son began to believe stories that General Dyer's troops lost their heads and opened fire—and continued to fire their machine guns into the dense and helpless crowd of Indians milling around in the restricted square.

'Massacre' is a word; but the thing of which it is the name is . . . is . . . well, it depends on your point of view. After long experience I found that there was an artist who could show me the beauty of a butcher's shop. I would not have noticed that the Little House in Delft was beautiful if Vermeer had not drawn my attention to it. So why is it that I remained blind to the beauties of a massacre at Amritsar or of the preservation of soldierly discipline even when provoked by the helplessness of a crowd?

What has all this got to do with your friend at Alfriston?

One day I was alone at The Gold Cross, a pub at Alfriston whose unpretentious appearance could not compete with the rival, wood-timbered elegance of The Star. Baudelaire's description of the useless glitter of a distant star and the unapproachable majesty of the beautiful woman, shows better than I could ever do the fundamental superiority of the comfort of The Golden Cross in contrast with the then fussy emptiness of The Star and its patrons. I walked to the beach and lay disconsolate and alone, lamenting the rocks and the seaweed, which made the possibility of a swim uninviting, and the lack of 'human face divine'. As if in response to my unspoken thought, a young man and an extremely beautiful young woman approached. "Hullo Wilfred! Whatever are you doing here?" It was the girl who I had grown used to thinking was my 'fiancée'. The word, with its fidgety quality of suburban and aristocratic gentility contrasted sharply with the storm of feeling in me. Before I could reply she had become aware of it and moved off on the supporting and possessive arm of the young man.

'None but the brave deserve the fair', and one thing I had learnt in war was that I was not—never could be—'brave'. When I had recovered my composure I moved along to the part of the beach where they were sitting. I apologized for my rudeness, saying I had been surprised and disconcerted. She offered me a small apple by way of sharing their lunch. I took it and moved off. They said they were moving further east along the coast; I returned to the company of my thoughts.

Later that day I was walking along the river back to my pub when I found myself caught up by the pair. No, they had changed their minds and were going to stop the night at Alfriston. I had their company. I was wearing plus-fours—a costume which I felt did not suit me and which seemed to be more than usually ridiculous and out of place. So was my state of mind.

The next morning was cool and fine. I stood outside my pub thinking of nothing in particular when 'he' came along. He struck me as a pleasant and unassuming fellow as he came up and started a conversation. 'She' arrived. As I write this account I am aware that it might be a confession made in the course of a police statement—I shall describe the crime later. "Where were you?" she asked, surprised that they had not seen me earlier. I said I had stayed at what was alleged to be a smugglers' inn, which I thought was less pretentious than the famous Star—"not so boarding-housey", I said, remembering the days of suburban Make-Believe in Stoke Newington before the flames of World War Two had brought poverty and dignity to the Capital of the British Empire and the World. "Oh no! It's not at all", was her 'correct' reply. I remained physically present, but I ceased to have any further conversation with her.

I am sure that must have been a terrible loss to her. No wonder you feel you are making a police report!

I cut short that week-end by making the transparent excuse that I had been recalled to London. I was haunted by that walk along the reedy path of the river. If I had had my service revolver with me I would have shot him. Then I would have shot her through the knee in such a way that the joint could not be repaired and she would have had a permanently rigid leg to explain to her future lovers. I would not give myself up because that would not be enough of a mystery to occupy the newspapers. But when in the course of ordinary routine enquiries they closed in on me I would make my report.

If I may say so, it sounds pretty dull.

Even if I had had my service revolver and ammunition—a most unlikely conjunction of events—I think I would have been deterred by that possibility. Who knows? Of course, in England you are not supposed to support your claims to masculine superiority by force—not unless you have a platoon of troops and an unarmed crowd on which to test your machine guns.

I doubt very much that a good journalist would think he could do much with a sordid little murder such as you visualized. What did *you do?*

Went back to Gower Street and misery. Now—

When is 'now'?

Say 1978 for convenience—I think humiliation is the price I paid for yielding great power to someone else. It seems that this is the cost in misery and suffering to any one person who surrenders power to another.

Always? Or only when the surrender is made without circumspection?

Two people who rush rhapsodically to the state of emotional bliss of perfect union pay in suffering for having evaded the toils of discovery of each other.

Reminds me of nothing.

Then try this: *She* took on a ready-made hero (certified genuine and authoritatively guaranteed) without the toil of discovering who or what *he* was. *He* took on a ready-made cosmetically guaranteed beautiful person without the toil of discovering what, if any, difference there is between a boy and a girl, a wife and a girl, a husband and a boy, a wife and a mother, or a husband and a father.

Don't be silly—how are they to find out? It's not in the schedule of any training course.

No, they find out the hard way by going to England to school, by not doing sexual things, by 'winning' military crosses, by becoming independent, twenty-one, earning their own living and 'free' to do whatever they like. It hurts. I took a—literally—hell of a time to discover it, and I didn't like hell or the long sojourn in which I was detained. And yet I am not Milton— and even he was just a Cambridge undergraduate who wrote Lycidas, backed the wrong side, although he thought it won a war, and—

Oh well, we all know about Milton, and who reads Paradise Lost *anyway?*

I do—thanks to Ruskin, another gifted, tiresome throw-out.

You might include Mohammed and Jesus and Moses. And while we are at it, why not God? He never got into a decent club or football team.

They do these things better nowadays by democratic election procedures.

Aren't you being sarcastic?

It's possible; I'm only human. Perhaps you ought to make allowances for God—He's only divine after all, poor...

Devil? Surely that's a contradiction in terms.

Only a contradiction in *terms*—articulate speech is in its infancy and has not reached a degree of refinement necessary for clear thinking.

Well, so far you have only got to medical school without having the slightest success with your genitalia, for all the numerous potential mates—male and female.

World War Two wasn't much more of a success than World War One.

Are you referring to personal, private, integer success? Or social, public continuum success?

Both. The progress is difficult to assess in view of the undetermined direction.

Ah! So Homo Sapiens has a bit to learn about Cosmic Navigation.

This particular Homo-not-so-Sapiens has. How the hell am I to get through Inter. B.Sc. with my lady-love being free to do just whatever she likes?

You will have to learn to do just what you don't like, when you don't like it, and whether the result is what you like or not. See the next fifty years.

I was incapable of being interested in what I now know to have been subjects which were of even greater relevance and importance to me than the subjects I failed to learn at Oxford, though they also, I find now—

When is—

(Don't interrupt; I'm thinking)—it would be useful if I could search through the debris of my mind, the ashy remnants of what once was a flaming fire, in the hope of revealing some treasure which would reconstitute a valuable piece of wisdom—a spark amidst the ashes that could be blown into a flame at which others could warm their hands.

What about your Inter. B.Sc.?

I got through by one mark—so I was told.

You must have been a master of the art of not quite falling off the fence.

It was extremely uncomfortable.

How do you think you and your girl-friend did in the combined assault on the Inter. Marital Sc. exam?

Failed—obviously.

You certainly did not get a Fellowship at Oxford.

I wouldn't even have dared to think of it.

Or the Headmastership of your old school.

Luckily for the school and for you.

I think it is just as well that there was a sexual barrier so that you failed to marry any of your boy-friends.

I do not remember any whom I would have liked to have as my husband—or parent to my children.

Any of your male colleague's spouses?

God forbid—

Perhaps He did.

I did not enjoy Inter. B.Sc., and getting through by one mark was only one aspect of a long experience of teetering along being a remarkably lifelike specimen of a bloody fool. Yet I think I remember, or imagine—I don't even now know which—that there was a time when I was not one.

When you got your DSO perhaps.

Don't be so ridiculous. I was never such a fool as not to know that if that sniper had aimed at me as skillfully as he did at Captain Edwards I would have been dead.

There were times when you were not obviously sensible; for example, when you left your tank—

It is difficult to relate being 'sensible' to taking part in war.

Or 'in love'.

Does anyone know what that is? God knows and He, as they say, won't split. Anyhow, I was not in a philosophical or contemplative mood, or I might have noticed that when we met again she was disappointed that I seemed to have got on very well without her.

You might also have noticed that she was only a young girl and not *a mature woman. Anyhow, how much longer are you going on with this extremely uninteresting and commonplace story?*

It was not commonplace or boring to me.

Well, you read it then.

It was very painful to me; there was no doubt about that part of the story.

It was a lover and his lass that o'er the green cornfields did pass.

Prithee pretty maiden will you marry me?
Hey, but I'm doleful, willow willow waley.
Nobody I care for comes a-courting—therefore Oh willow waley oh—
I think you've got it muddled up.

I don't mind if I have because I'm *not telling the story of my life. Those who want to write the story of their lives have a problem: that problem is not mine, and my problem is not theirs.*

I cared at one time what happened to the girl and felt it as my problem, but I was invited in no obscure language to mind my own business and told that her business was not mine. Here I am trying to tell the story of *my* business—part of which was the problem of existing.

6

THE 'analyst' to whom I had gone for 'cure' said it would require about twelve sessions to dispel the anxiety from which I was suffering after my scholastic and athletic failures at Oxford. As I could muster the requisite fee for twelve sessions by using the remainder of my army gratuity, I took the plunge. In due course I exhausted my resources for the twelve sessions so I borrowed from a colleague (as he now was but who before the war had been my history master) and, since he was a kindly man, my 'analyst', who allowed me to accumulate a debt. It was in the course of being 'analysed' that I had been sacked from my job, sacked by my extremely beautiful fiancée, and was well on the way to failing to get medically qualified also. The debts amounted to about £70 to my analyst and £30 to my colleague. The sum of £100 was truly terrifying to me in my parlous state; in contrast to my finances, the acquisition of a fund of failure seemed to be inexhaustible. So I stopped my attempts to be cured.

In this context it was very comforting to be offered a chance of curing an adolescent boy, the son of an army General, by using the same methods as had been—so far—unable to achieve the anticipated cure.

Who anticipated it—you or your analyst?

I don't know how much I believed it. I had half believed the surgeon's story that my torn cartilege would be fit for the Varsity Match. But I didn't consider that a half-belief, or even a half-cure, warranted my risking Oxford's chance to beat Cambridge, and accordingly told a disappointed Moresby-White that I could not be included in the team. I did not, however, tell the Dean of the Medical School that I was no good as a prospect for the UCH cup final team. After all, having a torn cartilege was not likely to stop me being a doctor so I do not consider myself at fault in being accepted as a medical student on the strength of my non-existent capacity as a rugger player.

My 'Feel it in the Past' analyst—

You have not explained this phrase.

He had a phrase which he used whenever the patient—myself in this instance—complained of some unpleasant occurrence. The theory was that some traumatic event in the patient's past life was 'repressed' and therefore caused him to have unpleasant sensations associated with the 'past' trauma but not related to the present in which he was living. As I contemptuously put it, "If your girl runs away with a rival today, don't worry, but feel it in the past." There is a kind of mad logic about it which was peculiarly convincing and impervious to my—then—critical capacity.

What about this infernal problem of Inter. B.Sc., learning anatomy and physiology, earning enough to pay £100 in debts, and not being sunk (without a trace of course) by your partner?

I could not find the answer.

So . . . you passed by one mark!

That is *not* funny: it may be psycho-analysis though. Anyway, Dr Feel-it-in-the-Past sent me the adolescent boy. I did not have much chance to tell him to feel it in the past because he dealt with *that* problem by not coming, telling his father he came regularly, and pocketing the fee which, though small, did at least defray his expenses in travel away from the General. It couldn't last: the General, smelling a rat, came to see *me.* It wasn't any good my telling him I was not a rat or to 'smell it in the past'. Another ghastly failure to add to my growing collection.

Didn't you have any *successes?*

I felt like the Indian student who is said to have added to his list of achievements 'Failed B.A.'. My ex-girl-friend's hostile "You seem to have got on very well without me", left me unable to reply, "Oh no, I can't get on without you", or, "Oh yes; I got on very well without you for years before I had ever heard of your existence." Yet I knew there was a right answer, and that I did not know what it was.

Do you mean you were unsure about its moral correctitude?

No. What added to the difficulty of the problem was that there was no moral doubt about its moral correctitude, but none the less the answer was wrong.

51 per cent seems to be your chance of success.

As a working indication it is not very helpful because it is not easy to distinguish between a score of 49 and one of 51.

At this period I became acquainted with Freddy John Poynton who was one of the chief physicians. I was, as a result of passing the Inter. B. Sc., entitled and even expected to present myself at his ward rounds. His comments on medicine, himself and his fellow learners were always pleasantly astringent. "The Vandenberg test of liver function", he said, "is extremely accurate. In cases of certainty it is always certain and positive; in negative cases it is negative; in doubtful cases it is doubtful." In other words, I thought, in real life it is useless. But in real life tests *are* useful as a way of appearing to support the existence of an impartial, scientific procedure on which one can rely as a substitute for one's own fallible judgment. The fallibility of my Self had by this time been amply demonstrated; nor was I able to feel any greater conviction about Selves other than mine. For example, Dr FiP had assured me I could never find another mate to equal 'her': this was certainly in accordance with my own opinion and clearly with the opinion of the Lady herself. But there was no available evidence to convince me that anyone, least of all myself, could fall back on my Self. There was no one else: I had tried God, but whenever I fell back on my faith in God I felt I was making a fool of myself and such religious experience as I had; there were 'Nigger' my prep school master, Chips, Chas, Bobby, and Sammy who could never understand why his dog, known to us boys as Sam after the Headmaster, would not answer to his proper name when called. Now I can see that the poor animal did not know his proper name any more than I did. As God had not been a great success, it was hardly surprising that the various human beings whom I had admired, adored and worshipped turned out to be inadequately equipped for the part I wanted them to play. Also, I seemed to lack the qualification to be an adequate human being even in the apparently lowly role of worshipping or adoring from afar. This made things difficult because the hospital, with whose wards I was now to become familiar, had a truly remarkable staff—Wilfred Trotter, Charles Bolton, Freddy John Poynton, Julian Taylor, Batty Shaw, Bill Williams, and He of the 'butterfly percussion', so remarkable because when he percussed a chest he did so with such delicacy that the unbelievers, including me, could not understand how something so ethereal as his palpations and percussions could yield any information at all. Still, he was Irish and I tried to believe that he shared with his race the quality of being 'fey'. Being 'fey' I understood to be a spiritual quality not quite holy but not quite devilish either. After one of these ethereal examinations he would draw us aside out of ear-shot of the patient, thus demonstrating the delicacy of his concern and arousing the patient's curiosity to a fever of impatience to hear what was being said about him. One of the physicians' clerks would be sure to pass it on later; I could not because I was not one of his clerks. But even if I had been, I could not have passed on his diagnostic summary, which was communicated in terms as delicate as his examination.

Charles Bolton was as earthy as—I shall call him MacWhitter—

was spiritual. But at least I knew what he meant, though I was not medically sophisticated enough to appreciate what he said. I was careful to carry out my clerkly functions to the best of my ability, as Charles—for all his easy-going manner and assumption of disillusioned devil-may-care—was not a person I felt disposed to be casual with in professional activities.

Wilfred Trotter was small and neatly but powerfully built. His strong hands had a beauty which could not by any stretch of the imagination be regarded as the product of a manicurist's cosmetic skill. I remember the near horror with which I saw him enter a skull with powerful blows of a mallet on the chisel he held. Such was his control that he could and did penetrate the hard bone and arrest the chisel so that it in no way injured the soft tissue of the underlying brain.

Once a week he saw, with his attendant dressers of whom I was one, new and old patients who came up to the hospital from their homes and work. Julian Taylor also had his out-patient clinic and it was therefore possible to observe the contrast in styles of two brilliant, world-famous (at that time) technicians at work.

Julian Taylor found it difficult to tolerate fools gladly. This was particularly noticeable to me from my centrally placed position of the fool. Now I would allow myself the favourable title of ignoramus rather than fool; I also think it wiser to regard the patient as ignorant rather than foolish—though of course he could be both—and I was in no position, in view of my knowledge of my history, to be in any way confident that *I* was not both.

This point had been penetratingly clearly brought home to me by my ex-girl-friend. I was aware of her sneering contempt when in one of my last talks with her—it was in the bustle of Trafalgar Square—I tried in tongue-tied confusion and humiliation to behave as if she should keep me as a suitor. I thought it most unfair that I should be so humiliated by her, and at the same time that I was blameworthy for being so contemptible. Later I understood these matters better, partly as a result of experiences such as those which I am describing when I compare Julian Taylor and Wilfred Trotter.

J. T. could not tolerate the response to his enquiry "What is your trouble?", "It's my kidneys doctor." "Kidneys! What do you know about kidneys!" (or liver, or stomach, or whatever other anatomical structure or physiological function to which the patient chose to refer). It offended both his medical knowledge and his sense of propriety. The patient, frightened at having given offence to such an eminent authority, would close up and volunteer no further suggestions lest a further storm be evoked.

Trotter, on the other hand, listened with unassumed interest as if the patient's contributions flowed from the fount of knowledge itself. It took me years of experience before I learned that this was in fact the case. When a patient co-operates so far as actually to present himself for inspection, the doctor from whom help is being sought is being given the chance of seeing and hearing for himself the origin of the pain. No need to ask, "Where does it hurt?"—though it would clearly be a comfort to have his query answered in a language that he understands. The anger that is so easily aroused is the 'helper's' reaction to an awareness that he does *not* understand the language, or that the langage that he *does* understand is not the relevant one or is being employed in a manner with which he is unfamiliar. Trotter's undisturbed friendly interest had the effect of eliciting further evidence from the patient; the fount of knowledge did not dry up.

It was said that when Trotter did a skin graft it 'took'; if Taylor did a skin graft—with equal or maybe even greater technical brilliance and accuracy—it did not take; the body rejected it; it was sloughed off. This I did not see, but that the story was told was itself significant of the impression that was created by the two men on their students.

Trotter's lectures seemed dull; there was nothing dramatic or spectacular about them. The reason for this lay partly in my own ignorance which precluded the pleasure that I might have obtained had I known enough about the matter on which he lectured, although when Elliot-Smith lectured on the brain I could see the brilliance of his spontaneous drawings on the board. Trotter did not draw such aids to comprehension but he spoke with an authority, a mastery of the subject which was unmistakable.

Oh, my God! Just as I was hoping to go to bed this ruddy woman has to come down the slope (not slippery) into Casualty. "Why do you have to come at midnight? Couldn't you have come earlier?" She is apologetic. She knows it was wrong not to come earlier, but she has three kids who had to be fed and as her husband has deserted her she has no one to leave them ... "Oh all right! All right! What's the trouble?" What a bloody nuisance these poor women are—why can't they marry faithful husbands? Who knows? Why does a skin graft take? Why does it slough off? The operation had been properly, technically performed. They were married in Church. but the marriage did not take, so now—no bed yet. I could yawn my head off. But if I go to sleep what dreams may come? Who is to be sure that they are 'only dreams'? As for this autobiography ... Truth? Or cosmetically acceptable fiction?

Do you mean, Mr Trotter, that I have to know what I am talking about? Do you think I might find a girl who would want to be married to me? And be a parent to our children? She might think I was brave; on the other hand she might not, and I don't like that much. Betty, pale-faced even against the unusual snow of Bournemouth, tried to believe the men were all right—my Colonel, my chiefs, and even my self. And for that I have never been able to exempt myself from cowardice. I didn't know. I didn't know—no, but I should have known.

7

THE operation was a simple one, not likely to present any difficulty to a really capable surgical technician. Clearly there would be no point in alarming the parents of the child in advising the operation for cleft palate. The anaesthetist was capable; she was also beautiful—no point in alarming anyone by causing them to question her cosmetic qualifications. They looked beautiful in the curriculum vitae. It was a beautiful curriculum vitae; it was also a beautiful day and the surgeon was in a good humour. He and his anaesthetist engaged in amusing banter as the operation proceeded with exemplary smoothness.

"I think her heart has stopped beating sir", said the House Surgeon.

"Good Lord!" said the surgeon. "Quick! When? ... Massage her heart!"

No good; no good. The child is dead.

No more. Quite spoilt our day. House Surgeon's job to tell the parents—there's been a slight mishap. As you would know—anyone would know—there was nothing technically wrong with the operation. Of course Wilfred Trotter wouldn't have known it was a fine day and just the time for a little harmless banter—he took things so seriously. He was a bad-tempered man; I even knew him be bitingly sarcastic about his extremely able theatre sister. "But Sister", he said, "I didn't ask you to answer back!"

Even Trotter made mistakes; I was not swearing when I clicked my tongue with vexation at not being able to grasp yet another Spenser Wells. Yet ... yet ... The operation was over and he was sewing up the wound. And I, and no one else in the relief at the completion of a tense and dangerous operation—not technically simple like a cleft palate—noticed that needle lying in the wound. Damn it! Why the hell should I risk getting half-murdered by opening my mouth? Simpler to let them find out in X-ray afterwards.

What a funny voice! Who is that talking in the theatre? That bloody fool again?

"Sir, there's a needle lying in the wound." Such a queer voice.

"Needle? Where?" Not at all funny voice—angry.

"There sir."

He picked it out and completed the sewing up.

"There", he said, handing me a piece of blood-stained thread, "that's what you want isn't it?"

I think I could have worshipped Trotter for that remark and gift. Not particularly witty or brilliant, but unmistakably said as only a great man could say it.

What about the mishap with the child?

All ended well by the House Surgeon telling the parents there had been a . . . misfortune. "Nothing serious?" asked the mother. No, no, not serious. Only your child is dead. They will get over it. Now—what about the body? Would they like the hospital to make the . . . ?

As the reinforcements entered Singapore harbour, Julian Taylor had to pack his kit as he was to be senior surgeon at the Military Hospital. It was time to land. Unfortunately two of the most powerful battle-cruisers in the world had just been sunk by Japanese dive-bombers; the decks were not armoured sufficiently powerfully to protect the magazines against that sort of suicidal attack. So two powerful insurances against the loss of Singapore had disappeared, and Julian Taylor, with the rest of the reinforcements, landed into captivity. No doubt Taylor was able to teach the Japanese surgeons a lot about the technique of surgery. Of course he would have the best para-medical services and most attentive surgical audiences during the hours of daylight; not much opportunity for banter because you never know if the Japs understand a joke. J. T.'s sense of humour I heard was also never the same again after the mishap of being delivered, thoroughly technically equipped but otherwise as right as rain, into the hands of the Japanese all waiting and anxious to learn.

And the sailors and soldiers?

Well, any survivors could make (Great) Britain fit for heroes to die for. The contestants in the Third World War will have to get on without the British Empire. But how was I to get on without anyone to advise patients to come to me? The adolescent boy was getting on; whether very well or not I do not know, but certainly without me. I would soon be licensed to practise medicine, but I knew virtually nothing about medicine and I was shortly to discover that the 'psycho-analysis' I knew was better suited to financial manipulation than the 'cure' of—souls? Can I minister to minds diseased? I was not capable of being any sort of parson. And the new problem which faced me was as unexpected as I now find it difficult to describe.

There was a practice, followed by certain people and strongly disapproved of on ethical grounds, of recommending patients to go to practitioners who consented to pay so much cash in return for each patient received. This method, known as fee-splitting, meant that a doctor who had achieved high position could make a very considerable income by sending patients who consulted him to one of these financially tied physicians or surgeons. The objection to this practice was of course that the patient would not be recommended to someone who would be most likely to know how to treat his ailments, but to someone who was willing to pay a percentage of his fees to the doctor first consulted. All the doctors with whom I associated were audible if not vociferous, in condemning such behaviour. It was accordingly something of a shock to me to find that Dr FiP expected me to pay him a percentage on every patient he recommended to me, and then and there proposed that I should enter into this business relationship with him.

"But Doctor," I said with all the naïvety and indiscretion of which my late Headmaster (now happily united with his Maker) had accused me when demanding my resignation, "isn't that fee-splitting?"

"Oh no, not at all", and he proceeded to make it clear to me, in ways that I regret not being able to make clear now, that this was not so.

However, though I may have had one other recommendation—thus proving the disinterested nature of his favours—our close collaboration wilted, dropped and died. I had learned that if I could not find some way of recommending myself to the favourable attention of some member of the universe of which I was a member, I would cease to be a member of anybody or anything at all.

I therefore rented a prestigious but sordid room in Harley Street and thereby launched myself on my first step as an artificial representation of what I hoped looked like a Harley Street Consultant. The consultants to whom I had become accustomed, with the exception of the Lord of the Butterfly Percussion, had seemed to me to be persons of substance. If I, as I hoped, was a person of substance, I had not so far discovered any substance of which I should be glad to be composed. I was a nothing. "Feel it in the past", I used to say. But anything that I felt, I *felt* in the present—and most unpleasant it was.

What were your feelings?

My analyst was a charming and intelligent man. I thought he was proposing a fee-splitting association; I was shocked. This could have been a non-conformist moral theory—like the others I had learnt or acquired or taken for granted in my suburban, Misses Evans-Cuff culture. "I know what *you* would like—run down to Spivey's for me and get me . . ." I did not like it any more than I would like to join a partnership, have paying patients and part with a percentage of the fees. Clearly I did not like to run errands even if I hadn't anything else to do—or anything I could say I *had* to do. I did not want to spend my time or my money in the way that *they* knew I would like. Using up a whole packet of Vim—that I *did* like. It would have been no good saying, "I know what *you* would like—for me to use a whole packet of Vim taking the enamel off your bath. You would love it!" No one had asked me if I would like to lay down my life for my country. For a long time I thought I would get away with it until it became impossible to be insensitive to the evidence that if I went on going into battle I would be killed.

My cousins—Marguerite, Herbert and Arnold—were not like my analyst or my suburb. They came from the suburbs: Blackheath, S.S.M.—School for the Sons of Missionaries. But although the difference was unmistakable, I could not say what it was. These cousins asked me out during one school holiday and gave me one glorious day of freedom from what I now know was a virulent, vigorous, overpowering culture of non-conformist Protestant cant. Marguerite had made a curry such as I had not tasted since I had left India when I was eight. Then they took me to see a matinée performance of *The Scarlet Pimpernel*. "Why does he say there are two damned spots of mud on his polished boots?" Herbert not only knew, but he didn't mind explaining. Trotter could not possibly help knowing I was a fool, but he was able to respect my feelings. I loved Marguerite and Herbert and Arnold and Trotter though I could never have dared to admit it. Today, thanks to greatly increased knowledge (psychoanalytic), everyone knows that I had a 'hetero-sexual, homo-sexual, gastronomic love' for my cousins. And that of course explains everything—except to me.

8

AND now this war—with Germany of course. Ridiculous. Why is it that nobody did anything about it while I've been busy getting qualified? Well, thank goodness Mr Chamberlain had the sense to go and *see* Hitler and it has all been settled.

So I could go for two or three weeks to Church Farm, Happisburgh, in Norfolk, with a party of friends including actor John Glyn Jones and actress Betty Jardine. That at least was a success: Glyn Jones was extremely amusing; Betty Jardin, whom I had seen in *The Corn is Green* as Bessy Watty and also at the Players Theatre, was not so amusing, nor as attractive as I had expected, but was likeable. She was obviously a very fine actress. Nuisance about Hitler though.

I went on from Happisburgh to the south of France, passing through Monte Carlo which was on the route but otherwise uninteresting; nice petunias in the central square seemed to fill the neighbourhood with their glorious odour. But it was not sufficient to screen the less appealing stench of Hitler and Nazi Germany. It was easy to believe that the stink of the corpse of Imperial Germany mingled with the stink of decay from Imperial Britain was what the athletic perfume of post-war Oxford had failed to disguise in 1919. This was twenty years later and I still could not get the smell of Glory out of my hair. Roquebrune and its orange blossom, a walk to Monte Carlo, a good dinner and not very expensive vintage champagne, the soothing rhythm of the surf below my window—it was *very* agreeable. But I had no company except my thoughts, and twenty years had not been long enough to establish these with sturdy roots. I cared for nobody enough to form a dense, impenetrable barrier against ... but surely I could not be called up to join the dis-armed forces of Very Great Britain? Once you have learnt, have been really taught that you are a coward, no amount of official certification by the highest authorities is any more use than the first aid bandage slung across the gap where Kitching's chest wall should have been; it could not render invisible his heart beating away his life.

I would be called up or volunteer for the medical services. The not-so-glorious RAMC...Stretcher bearers! Stretcher bearers! Coming sir! Coming. Nice bit of water skiing today sir! Put you right in a moment! No thanks; I can swim anyhow. What about a nice Second Class in Finals sir? Or a Rugger Blue? The Nazis are on the verge of collapse; my sister who works for a fellow whose father owns a mine in the Ruhr, she knows for a fact that they *could not* ... Yes, thank you very much. I feel fine.

Time to get back to Harley Street. A nice cushy job in Hobart House perhaps.

Hobart House? Never heard of it.

It's just near Buck House.

You mean Buckingham Palace?

That's out of date now. Democracy has broken out. Oh no, not National Socialism; that's only in Germany.

I returned and gave my landlord notice as I thought there was no point in paying rent for a consulting room I could not use. My landlord was anxious that I should leave the Gordon Russell heater in place. So was I. It was utterly ineffectual, but it gave off a warming coppery glow—that is if you could not tell the difference between hot and cold but could use your eyes for purposes of self-deception. Not *now*—feel it in the past. So, if you did not like the present you could build yourself a beautiful cocoon and warm your hands and any remnants of a heart in the expensive cosmetic achievements of Gordon Russell. Yes, he could keep it as part payment for rent and the earlier termination of my lease.

I joined the army. As a major.

So you went on where you left off.

Not quite. The bilge had increased and what I thought was courage was only froth. I do not know what had happened to the spark of sincerity which had been blown into a flame by Marguerite, Herbert and Arnold. The years of this Second World War hardly bear being thought about. The froth, the bilge, the sanctimonious cant, submerged but never storm-tossed and therefore waiting, waiting unimpaired to take control. Surely, I thought, there must be some remnant of decency left? Or was it all 'feel it in the past—it will pay you just as it paid me'?

What had happened to the spark of sincerity?

Just before the war I found I could not stand the 'feel it in the past' conspicuous consumption of erosive and corrosive glory. In spite of being warned that psycho-analysts were a lot of Jews, foreigners and psychopaths—most un-English in fact—I went to see John Rickman. In those days he was blunt-spoken and frighteningly impatient of cant. I liked him; I agreed, with great misgivings, to start analysis. To my surprise his interpretations appeared to me to be reminiscent of common sense; they reminded me of real life. I was astonished because common sense did not seem to be grand enough. Rickman's interpretations and his behaviour stirred up the dead embers of the pile of rubbish which was all that I could see of *Sesame and Lilies*, *Lycidas*, Colman's sunny study, Gilbert and Sullivan, 'days of fresh air in the rain and the sun', Oxford University, University College London, Jack Drummond ... ashes ... ashes ...

Drummond and his wife and child, on holiday in a caravan in the south of France, had been murdered. The trial was a farrago of lies which were so non-sensical that the successive declarations, "Now, I will tell you what really happened", could have been the refrain of a musical comedy—but for those three corpses. Rickman, however, seemed to be familiar with murder and that it could occur in France and England as well as in Soviet Russia, where he had lived.

I thought Rickman liked me. (Ah ha! I thought so—counter-transference!) But there was some kind of emotional turbulence, with its high and low pressure areas, which extinguished the analysis as far as Rickman and I were concerned. It stopped; though not before it had also extinguished any spark of respect that might have been entertained for me by my pre-psycho-analytic colleagues, and before I had penetrated far enough to be independent.

I was ordered to report to Western Command. So, with my travel voucher, up to Western Command I went. I found my way to the Medical Headquarters and was civilly informed that I should really have gone to Aldershot. "But ... well, you know how things are in the army", the Colonel said before dismissing me. Fuming at the waste of time and money before recalling to my comfort that it was not now *my* time and money because I was being paid, I caught an express which happily was just leaving for London, rang up Betty Jardine and had a very pleasant dinner at Quaglino's before I 'proceeded'—in the army I never 'went' anywhere—to Aldershot the next day. As I remember it now, that was the last time I experienced any sense of amusement for many years. Frustration, futility, anger and humiliation were commonplace not only to me and Betty, but to the society of which I was a member.

At Aldershot perfunctory squad drill was carried out as if it were, and indeed as it was, totally irrelevant. The title of the Corps, we were told in a lecture, was the R for Royal, A for Army, M for Medical, C for Corps. The regular officer who was lecturing said they did not want any such indiscipline as had led, in the 1914-18 war, to the RAMC becoming known throughout the Army as the 'Rob All My

Comrades'. Well, I thought, thank God they learnt something in the First War. There were brave men in the medical services just as, I had very good reason to know, there were cowards in the combatant regiments. I likewise had learnt that I did not want to become infamous as a coward any more than I wished to be famous for being what I knew I was not. And now I was supposed to be part of the psychiatric service—dealing with the psyche. Not the soul exactly—that was the job of the Chaplain's Department—just the psyche if you know what I mean (because I don't). We had to tell the authorities if the man who was offering himself, or was offered by somone else, as suitable to lead his fellows in war had the right kind of character (soul, disposition, super-soul, id, ego, or super-ego?) for the job. The physicians went into the physical qualification that presented itself; the bodies and minds of the selectors were assumed to be adequate. The only one about whom I had any private information was myself, and I could safely say that I knew *I* did not want to go into any battle.

At first I was not engaged in choosing officers; nobody gave me any orders other than that I was to report for duty at Craigmile Bottom Hospital. Nobody there knew what to do with me so I was put in charge of 'shell-shocked' patients.

The first one of these was Polish, could speak no English and was said not to be getting on in the army. With him came another Pole as translator; but he could not speak English either. The interpreter was a man of predominantly cheerful disposition and was clearly ready to co-operate. However, by tapping his forehead, and similar signs, he made it clear that his compatriot was mad. With some difficulty, and the remnants of the French and German I had learnt at school, I explained that I wanted to know what the patient was saying. This put my interpreter in a quandary: he tried hard to explain to me that the poor patient was 'mad', 'dotty', 'balmy', and therefore that he was talking nonsense and there was no point in his repeating to me what he was saying. However, he humoured me enough for me to gather that the patient had been in Warsaw and the Nazis ... the Nazis ... At this point his sense of humour overwhelmed him and he burst into uncontrollable laughter so I was never able to join in the joke about my patient and the Germans in Warsaw—beyond its being excruciatingly funny. While he wiped tears of laughter from his eyes and tried to adjust to the further hilarity of my taking this crazy man's statement seriously, the patient himself sat looking at the interpreter with undisguised disgust, and at me as if to find out how long he had to participate in the trio. After a while the interpreter tried to control his mirth, but as soon as he managed to listen to the patient his sense of humour became too much for him. He excused himself saying that he had never previously had the experience of listening to mad men and consequently had not realized that they were so funny. I began to be afraid that the possibility of having such an amusing life would lead him to take up training to become a psychiatrist himself. As I had to do a ward round I seized the opportunity to end the 'consultation'.

The hospital authorities had no idea what I was supposed to do any more than I had. But this state of affairs was not regarded with equanimity by Western Command who saw no reason why I should be treated any differently from any other medico with the rank of major posted to them for duty. However, I understood that in fact I was to be transferred to the hospital that was nearer to Western Command Headquarters so that I could have access to the Highest Authorities and could thereby bring my influence to bear. I do not think Western Command wanted to have any influence borne on them by anyone; I had the curious fantasy that if the Germans had by any chance landed in Western Command they would have been defeated by the sheer inertia of the troops of which it was composed—and I myself was no exception to the prevalent lethargy.

Ultimately I obtained a pass to visit all the various units, including a Royal Navy establishment. The regular naval officer in command had been a Chief Petty Officer and had risen from the ranks. It must be remembered that an officer, RN, was traditionally no sailor but a gentleman: an officer who was a Royal Naval Volunteer Reservist was a ranker and neither a gentleman nor a sailor—like the Mercantile Marine, ex-sailors but no gentlemen. This commanding officer, whom I like very much, seemed to feel his position keenly; it soon became clearer to me what kind of difficulty he had to face. His wife, whom I also liked, had no problems as far as gentle birth was concerned, but . . . she had married a man who had risen from the ranks. She had therefore lost caste and had become, like my dear ayah, an untouchable.

The WRNS, unlike the ATS, was not under the same disciplinary code; there was therefore no military crime with which a Wren could be charged if she chose, as did one of them in this camp, the occasion of a ceremonial parade to cock a snook at the Camp Commanding Officer. With all the traditions of naval discipline behind him, and all the solid and gentlemanly traditions of privilege in front, the poor Commandant was at a loss. No Kings Regulations, no Debrett to be his guide; he had met his Trafalgar. Lord Nelson could do nothing for Lady Hamilton, and where Nelson failed it would be hardly fair to expect the Commandant to succeed. Besides, the Wren, unlike Lady Hamilton, was on the other side: the Commandant thought that a Wren officer would have to cope with the unusual Wren, private, able-seawoman. Poor man; he was glad to talk to me because he was so unused to finding someone who wanted to listen. Luckily the problem was no part of my psycho-job—psycho-analysis? psycho-therapy?

Robert Bridges, although he was Poet Laureate, had to dare to be a poet and take the risk of finding that he was not one, that poets are born—not made. He had good reason for knowing that there were such creatures because of his contact with Gerard Manley Hopkins who *was* a poet but was never made Poet Laureate. Poets Laureate are made, not born: I was made a psycho-analyst, but it soon became clear that I had not been born one. I could not imagine what I was supposed to be or do on the tour on which I was engaged when I met the British Lion whose non-existent tail was being twisted by the insignificant Wren. I went on with my tour—of which I knew no more than I knew of the ward round I engaged on as an escape from the hilarious Pole and the mad survivor from Warsaw.

Betty and I visited a unit in which the officers and men were rehearsing a variety show. One item included the popular song, 'Roll Out the Barrel'; they could not get it right. Betty told them to keep the time constant but halve the amount of action they were trying to cram into the time available for the words; they took the advice and the entire performance sprang into life. The unit and its C.O. were pleased and grateful; some of it overflowed into being glad that I, the Command Psycho-Whatnot, should come again.

On another visit the commander of the unit and his wife were kind enough to ask us to lunch. It was most successful—and amusing. The wife was very envious of Betty's curl of white hair which showed up against the background of dark brown. This, it appeared, was then most fashionable so Betty was in the height of the vogue, but lucky enough to be natural and not a cosmetic cheat.

Our hostess said she used to be able to sing once. When she essayed a few notes it was to demonstrate that her voice had now gone. "But", she added defiantly, "I could sing once." She was in fact Lottie Collins who had starred in *The Maid of the Mountains.* I asked if she regretted the Old Days. "No! Once I vowed I would be rich, I would marry a lord, and I would marry for love. I have done them all—so why should I regret?" She did look enviously, laughingly at Betty's hair; she knew that Betty was in *The Corn is Green*, but her envy had the laughter in it which was also friendly.

9

What about this Command Psychiatrist job?

I had to get on with my command performance, so we did not dally over much but moved on to the hospital where all was well organized and miserable. I asked one man what he was doing. He was doing "Occupational Therapy". This sounded as if it were something similar to what *I* was supposed to be doing; 'therapy' at least sounded familiar although I had no idea what my 'occupation' was.

"Yes, but what are you *doing?*"

He seemed sheepish as he said he was sewing a doll's dress. I looked at his steel helmet, his rifle and bayonet and other kit; it was all laid out in meticulously correct order. There was nothing wrong with that military hospital; nothing wrong with the 'military' part of it anyhow.

"Do you use these"—I pointed to his helmet and rifle—"for sewing dolls' clothes?"

He looked puzzled and I checked myself. After all *he* could hardly be held responsible for his equipment. And for me to press the point would have seemed to be verging on sarcasm. Anyhow, what was I doing with my military insignia? Loafing around Western Command?

At my next unit the commanding officer suggested we should take a stroll together. He would bring his gun because he might be able to augment the mess rations if he shot some pigeons.

"But they are cunning beggars I can tell you. If I were to point my cane at them they wouldn't mind in the least. Yet if I point my gun—or even carry the thing—you can be sure they won't wait to see. But they'll be around again immediately I go into the next field."

Pigeons know the difference between a gun and a walking stick; they would not be impressed by a social symbol of officer's rank—not enough to fall down dead, though I have known a partridge with chicks trail an apparently wounded wing away from its brood. In the mean time what was I to do to justify my rank and prestigious title of 'Command Psychiatrist'? Theirs not to do but die; theirs but to command and fly.

J. R. Rees came to see me. He wore brigadier's insignia so I thought I could put my problem to him. He was an old friend of mine so I did not stand on formality. Neither did he; he made it clear to me how extremely successful they had been in getting the notice and support of the Army Commander. Had I seen the Army Commander? "Good God! What the hell could I say to the Army Commander even if I got an interview?" The mere idea! But the others had 'sold' the Matrix Test which was simple and effective and had been taken up with enthusiasm by the Army Commander.

Nobody, least of all myself, could have been surprised when my old friend had me removed to a lesser post where I would be more in my element. So, in a week or two I found myself and Betty driving away from Western Command to the Area Command at York. I was angry and hurt. What else poor Rees could have done I do not know and did not much care. I had got the sack. Betty must have been trying to believe that she had not made a terrible mistake in marrying a bad-tempered failure; I likewise was not in a frame of mind in which I wanted to admit even the possibility that this could be true.

A miserable journey. "Don't snatch!" she said in response to my impatient gesture to look at the map. I was rude; and anxious. Eventually we stopped for the night. Was it Bosworth? Or another scene of someone's Civil War victory? How was it possible to remain so ignorant of the history in which I had been alleged to have an Honours degree? It certainly did not illuminate that bit of history in which I was participating by driving my car from Chester to York.

The two colonels to whom I was subordinate were as civil as their station in life called on them to be. But in war there is no particular reason for joyful anticipation of the prospect of prolonged co-operation. They suggested a billet in Whip-ma Whop-ma Gate. No, they didn't know why it was called that. I was made aware that that was the kind of idiotic remark, a display of irrelevant curiosity typical of a psycho-analyst—or more exactly of me, the Elephant's Child, one who does not learn for all its questions. Betty was as curious as I was, but she too learnt not to ask silly questions; there was a war on and no one could waste time on such—

How was York Cathedral? Had they arrested the ravages of the death-watch beetle?

York Minster couldn't be cared for in wartime.

What about Beverley Minster?

There was no time to visit those old sites. And luckily for us all, the two ancient Britons and I did not have to do any business together. I was to visit the 11th Armoured Division and its General

Hobart. This took me a long way out of York.

After reporting to Divisional Headquarters I went to see the Colonel of the first unit on my list. I entered and saluted. There was something vaguely familiar about . . . he reminded me of . . . Yes! His name was Willis. I had just been awarded the DSO and was talking to a fellow near Merlemont Plage. He was upset because he had just been invalided out of the Navy for defective eyesight, which was considered to be good enough for a commission in Tanks. Land ships were no use to him however; the Royal Navy was all that mattered.

He didn't recognize me but it was the same young Willis that I knew. Last time he had felt at home because I had at least a week's acquaintance with the Royal Naval Barracks at Chatham: this time it was I who felt pleased because I knew he thought highly of me and I was feeling the need for recognition.

I explained that the idea was to get rid of any soldiers with poor ability who therefore would not be likely to make good Tank soldiers. I added with emphasis that I did not back the results of a Matrix Test against the seriously considered view of an officer about his own men. He seemed relieved; he suggested I fix up details with his adjutant. So I felt I could venture an excursion into informality.

"The last time we met I was in the 5th Battalion", I said.

He looked up in surprise. "Bion!" he exclaimed with the relief—which was mutual—that must have been experienced when Crusoe and Man Friday met; like the shadow of a great rock in a thirsty land.

Is there any desert such as a sojourn amongst non-combatants?

Only once more, before I said goodbye to military service at the end of the war, did I have such relief. The farewell to non-combatant experience did not, and could not, bring me relief, but I did not realize that it might be possible to know too much; the dose has to be regulated in accordance with the degree of stamina or resistance the soul can command.

I am: therefore I question. It is the answer—the 'yes, I know'—that is the disease which kills; it is the Tree of Knowledge which kills. Conversely, it is not the successful building of the Tower of Babel, but the *failure* that gives life, initiates and nourishes the energy to live, to grow, to flourish. The song the sirens sing, and always have sung, is that the arrival at the inn—not the journey—is the reward, the prize, the heaven, the cure.

What about Colonel Willis?

Oh! Of course. "That's right. The same. Merlemont wasn't it?" Better not ask him about being a regular colonel in command of a cavalry regiment (armoured, as they call it, but the only armoured part of it that I had noticed was the state of mind).

"I was seconded to the Cavalry—used to be the Yeomanry—to give them a stiffening of regular officers."

Privately, I don't think you are rigid enough Willis—too much of the sea about you. "How do you like the Cavalry?"

"Better than Infantry, but they say ridiculous things like 'his tank was shot from under him' when they mean his tank was knocked out."

Or his Navy was knocked out when they thought they had only got rid of a keen young lad for defective sight.

"Of course they don't like Hobart much." (So I had noticed.) "He is at heart an engineer and when he inspects one of his battalions, instead of doing it properly like a regular cavalry officer would, he puts on overalls and gets under a tank with a spanner."

"Yes, I can imagine they might hate that."

"And what made you take to medicine?"

"That's a long story—I hardly know myself. I don't like this war much."

"I don't think Hobart does either—wants to be at the Front. So did I, but there was hardly a front to be at."

"The Boche were a bit too mobile for the Maginot Line."

"The Maginot Line wasn't mobile enough."

"Like our old tanks."

"Oh yes. Now the old top speed of 4 m.p.h. is about the lowest they go."

"Have you got Whippets, or the heavy tank we had in the 5th Battalion?"

"We haven't either. There are only one or two tanks—enough for Hobart to inspect."

There'll always be an England—unarmed, betrayed, 'bitched, buggered and bewildered' was the slogan. Am I not supposed to be one of the Governing Classes? What for? Full Blues at games of one sort or another? Guzzling? Gourmet meals? Decorations? What, me?! Should I have been agitating for arms for the Armed Forces—tanks, aeroplanes, ships? No. No, just feel it in the past. Support the Establishment. And as things have been, so they remain. Does it matter who 'governs' England, Europe, Africa, the World? Or 'quis custodiat custodes'?

"I'm supposed to be seeing the General at lunch time so I had better get off. What's he like?"

"He's a very good sort, but has put the back up the Powers-that-be and he is fed up because he can't get employment abroad. As he doesn't believe the Germans will land here, and nor do the Cavalry, he doesn't see any point in fiddling around with tanks which are out of date anyway."

"So they think horses would be more up to date? Or more picturesque?"

"I shouldn't ask him if I were you. He's pretty prickly and the war is a sore subject with him. Well, good luck—have a nice lunch. I doubt it though—they have an awful Mess; and Hobart, unlike the rest of his staff, doesn't care what he eats."

When I had walked and thought my way to HQ, I had still not digested what I had learnt so far.

"Ah! So you're the new psychiatrist. I don't want any mental defectives—I need intelligent people for my unit!"

"Yes sir. That is the point of these tests."

"Matrix? I know what they are supposed to show, and most psychologists I have met seem to be pretty intelligent. They don't always, starting with myself, seem to be particularly wise though. Come on—say something intelligent."

"I am ready to start testing at once."

"Good. Fix it up with the units."

"Of course tank crews have to be more than simply intelligent sir."

"I don't want any half-wits. The crews have to be intelligent."

"Certainly sir. But . . ." I wasn't doing very well. 'But me no buts' seemed to loom as the possible outcome of this talk. I decided not to risk getting involved in a conversation about Minds and wise agricultural labourers.

The meal having left my hunger unappeased and my misgivings augmented, I set out. There was no hope, and I harboured none, of any of the friendliness and co-operation that I had received from Willis. His was in fact a regiment in which the privates were mostly men of good education and I had reported to Willis that I saw no reason for not leaving good alone. Not so Hobart.

"What? You don't think any transfers necessary?" he bristled. The mere fact that I had reported so favourably aroused his suspicions. It was clear that he had anything but a favourable impression of his Division. I could see that though I might not recommend transfers, there was no difficulty about finding someone who wanted *me* transferred. The infantry battalion had far the best results and for once I thought the tests did not conflict with the impression that I received in interview. Hobart did not mind having intelligent infantry, but he was unshaken in his dissatisfaction with the intelligence of the cavalry.

And now for a meeting of the Command psychiatrists under the chairmanship of *the* Army psychiatrist (civilian). For me the highlight of this parade of our massed intelligence was one report: 'When the cavalry had horses, if the horse had a mental age of five and the rider a mental age of two, the respectable total could be assessed as a mental age of seven. But if the rider has a mental age of two and his mount is an inanimate piece of machinery, the combined mental age remains two. And this is not enough.'

This seemed to me to be an observation which was both entertaining and illuminating. It also came near to compensating for the exercise of compulsory attendance at a Command Conference. I cannot believe that the discussions I heard had any relevance to the selection of troops for battle or the selection of privates for training as officers. It was too late: fighting men and their leaders have to be grown. If the aim is to grow food should one not select the conditions which would be most conducive to the growth of the crop which is desired? It is not scientific to say, "Let there be land" and then, "Let there be peanuts." If one has land it would seem to be wise to experiment—to find out what would be likely to grow on that land. If the land appears to be ideally suited for the growth of a Wehrmacht, whoever owns that land will have an advantage over a land that is suitable for growing thinkers, or poets, but not soldiers. If the land is surrounded by sea and the proportion of land to water is correct, then a similar advantage would seem to accrue to the aim of growing sailors or a Royal Navy.

Can we recognize the minimum conditions necessary for the growth and nourishment of a population of sailors, airmen, poets? Or will they decay and die leaving only a shell, as the accepted rules for a poem might stifle rather than protect the growing germ of thought? The pre-Islamic ode, with its almost obligatory description of the camping site and its previous occupants, hardly seems to afford the minimum conditions necessary for the growth of Bach's Brandenburg Concertos, or Keats's 'Ode to a Nightingale', or an Impressionist painting.

Excuse me—don't you know 'there's a war on'?

Just the thing for poets! Arjuna, don't argue! Krishna knows best!

10

CLIFFORD Scott and Rickman both suggested that I should be posted to Northfield Military Hospital to take charge of the Military Training Wing. Lt. Colonel Pearce had agreed to put up with the consequences. He, like Rickman, Scott and myself, was an amateur medical soldier; he knew nothing about it but his badges of rank gave the impression that he did. I was still suffering from the DSO that had been inflicted, with my collusion, on me: the Senior Psychiatrist was suffering from having to appoint officers to the Shell-shock (as it was called) Hospital. None of us knew what shell-shock was or even if it existed outside the imagination of soldiers like me and Sergeant O'Toole who had to cope with the 'dumb insolence' of the little board-school slum-dweller, Allen, who had been considered to be just the stuff that heroes are made of, coming from a land fit to be loved by slum-dwellers who would want to die for it. Many thousands did not sing, 'Land of Hope and Glory', but 'Oh my, I don't want to die, I want to go home.'

Well, there it was: Military Training Wing, Northfield Military Hospital. All yours, Major Bion, DSO, Legion of Honour. Just the thing you would like to do, you Vim-wasting, bath-scrubbing, bloody little Oxford University Darling. If only I had a nice disposition like the little dog at Windsor Castle who had learnt that he would get a sweet biscuit if he lay on his side, I too would wag my tail and there would be no trouble.

I went to the programme room. Betty had gone back to London as the cast was touring with *The Corn is Green;* London hardly seemed the place for theatrical entertainment while the bombs were dropping. The chart showed all the possible activities available for soldiers who were being 'rehabilitated', that is to say, those who were on the journey to return to their units, cured—of what? Their love of fighting for their country? Love of the privileged darlings of Oxford? Or love of the Military Training Wing? Perhaps I should find out. But this is thirty-five years later and all I have acquired are a few more questions. 'No doubt but ye are the people and wisdom shall die with you.' Job was a sarcastic old devil; no wonder he was never popular.

I was impressed by the chart—the number of facilities, the actual administrative feat of time-tabling. I wondered just how effective these therapeutic activites were. It seemed late to be arranging these facilities *after* war had broken out and the men who were supposed to be fighting it had, supposedly, 'broken down'. Nevertheless I presumed that titles of centres such as 'Engineering Workshop', 'Carpentry Workshop', 'Art Workshop' had a meaning. I found three or four privates languidly waving dusters at the windows. They were not saying, "Goodbye".

In the days when 'Art thou weary? Art thou languid?' together with 'Summer suns are glowing' were my favourite hymns, I was depressed; I thought that I would become depressed if I saw much more of Northfield Military Hospital. I asked them what they were doing. "Orderly duty, sir." I suggested they should wave goodbye to the windows and come with me to see what the rest of the hospital was doing.

I have already described the experience of Northfield Hospital elsewhere.[1] Now that I write an autobiography I can be frank about how it feels to have been, once, a participant, and now a *laudator temporis acti*. Predominantly it is a matter of regret that an opportunity to achieve something valuable was precluded by being petty. Pearce could not have been expected to know any better and he needed help. So did Rees. It is therefore hardly surprising that they blundered. I could have helped them to avoid the worst blunders. But by stressing their blunders and indeed behaving in a way that made it clear that I would get them into further trouble, I deprived them of help and contributed to their making further blunders. About my Self I knew very little; about Pearce and Rees I knew nothing. It was like the relationship between my crew and myself and the forty tons of useless steel sinking fast below the mud of Hill 40; the Staff should have known about weather and ground conditions on Hill 40 in August.

How?

By asking their Intelligence Officer.

How would he know?

By being chosen for the job because he was intelligent. Clough Williams Ellis was very intelligent; that is why he asked me where I thought the subsoil turned to the aluvial. How the hell should *I* know?

[1] 'Psychiatry at a Time of Crisis', *Journal of The British Psychological Society*, Vol. XXI, 1948.

You had been taught all about the Flood in Scripture; in Geography you had learnt about subsoil from Becker Shaw.

I did not like Becker Shaw. Anyhow, I didn't know that I would one day owe my life to paying attention to floods and things. And I was too frightened that a 5.9 Howitzer shell, or even a 9.2 would land on my tank just as one had laid a pill-box on its side.

What about Pearce and Co.?

It's too long a story to go into all that now. Pearce told Rees, and Rees did not need any telling, that it was dangerous to have people as 'intelligent' as Rickman and me around because either we should blow up the Military Training Scheme (and the whole of Army Psychiatry), or one of the Big Guns would fire at us, and they—Pearce or Rees—would get hit.

So: what happened?

Rees had us posted off to where we could do no harm. So I shall never know what would have happened if privates in the Training Wing had caught the habit of asking questions or having opinions of their own which they might be able to hear in the silence of the sleep time when their fancies could become free to roam like the wind. In fact I think that some of the bees may have escaped from my bonnet.

I took the opportunity of meeting Betty on my way through London. She had by this time become more reconciled to the fact that I usually got the sack when my presence became obtrusive. Lunch was gastronomically pleasant—at Scott's—but both of us were simmering and therefore capable of boiling over. In less pictorial language, we considered the possibility of accepting an invitation to dine with Buchanan Smith who was in overall charge of the Military—in contrast with Medical—appointments in Officer Selection. So, we could have exposed the financial chaos of Northfield, and the mental chaos of Rees and Pearce which was responsible. But ... but ...

Disloyalty?

No. Any Scot who had 'Smith' tacked on to his name was pretty sure to have rebellion in his veins from the days of 1644. And anyhow, the organization that Rees and one or two amateur soldiers had built up was a structure that was more meritorious than evil—or so we thought. It is curious to reconsider past happenings in the light of the experience which, presumably, should have led to an accumulation of more knowledge, and to find that in matters which are basic the inadequacy remains; but the awareness of the one domain that lies unknown, undiscovered, can bring fresh poignancy to the discrepancy.

I duly 'proceeded' to my new posting which was in a suburb known as Selhurst. The commander of the unit was the youngest brother of a Field Marshal. As he was also a regular soldier, a guardsman, he was not intimidated by the machine of which he was a part, or by the latest of the 'temporary gentlemen' that he had temporarily inflicted on him. His easy-going ability to take life as he found it, without any urgent compulsion to reform it or the people in it, struck me as a welcome change from the psychiatric and not at all gentlemanly pyrexia in which I had been living for the last few years.

Betty, now no longer on tour with her company, was again acting to full houses in London and living with old friends in Pont Street, not far from Sloane Square, where a dilapidated sign indicated that the cinema was OOL, LEAN AND UMFY—the eliminated C reminded me of the village in Norfolk known as Larling. She was able once or twice to visit me at Selhurst and shared with me a liking for my amusing and intelligent Colonel. She became pregnant and we looked forward to the day when we should have a child. There also seemed a chance that the war would not last much longer.

I was interviewing officers who had been liberated by the Eighth Army from their captivity after the surrender at Tobruk. One had heard me lecture in the days when I was a War Office Selection Board psychiatrist.[1] "I don't remember what you said, but it was very amusing." Another found it very difficult to reconcile himself to the fact that he had surrendered. I discussed it with him and said it must be very difficult to know what to do when you have no time to think. I had never forgotten that Asser did *not* surrender and was shot through the heart. We, who are left, grow old—Asser did not. "After all", I said, "if you had been killed the Army would be an officer short and you could not escape or be freed to do more." Even now we should have to debate for a long while to decide what would be the intelligent thing to do.

Even then, there is the problem of what would be the wise thing.

I interviewed some four hundred officers who had been prisoners of war—presumably on the grounds that they needed rehabilitation. Later I learnt that they had not been shell-shocked or demoralized or forced into an impasse (such as I had experienced when I lay

[1] He interviewed 1,400 men between March 3 and August 6, 1943. The notes he wrote on every one, varying in length from a few lines to a whole page, remain unpublished. He bound them together in a book of almost three hundred pages, many of which are stained by the water used to extinguish fire bombs on the roof of the house in Pont Street during air attacks on London.

beneath a tin roof watching a piece of mud swinging rhythmically at the end of a straw each time a shell burst) but that each one had reacted according to his own nature. Many years later I heard a psychiatrist—who had not been to Vietnam or any other front—state that all those who had been taken prisoner had been 'brain-washed'. 'Washed in the blood of the Lamb' seems less revolting and improbable as a cleaning material, but no less unilluminating.

I take it that someone felt 'better' because there was a psychiatrist ('me', God help me!) available to see that they needed help. All the poor, unprivileged inhabitants of the Military Training Wing had similarly been subjected to a dose of 'Me plus Rickman', and Northfield 'minus Rickman and Me'. I hope they all felt better and are now 'fit to be heroes' in the Third Instalment (nuclear fission phase) of the War to End War. From what the physicists say it may well achieve that end. "These are fascinating times we live in my dear Bion", as an elderly acquaintance used to say to me. I hope it will be an equally fascinating time to die in.

Shortly after this the Authorities decided that the Western Front required the presence of my Colonel and his unit. I did not find out why, but by this time my contemporaries must have realized it was no good asking me questions such as, "What are you doing in Selhurst?" (or Brussels, or Cambrai, or Timbuktoo had I been sent there).

Betty had to make her last journey on her own, telling herself her last bedtime story about two nice men who were really being very brave and so considerate and kind. One of them was her husband, and I still cannot help hoping that she was not deprived of the comforting lie that he was really a man and a hero, and not just an artificial representation of a man stuck up in the show-case of a universe signifying nothing and tricked out with psycho-analytic dummies intended to fool the psycho-analytic church into believing that there are real souls that require to be humanized. What if there *were* thoughts and feelings and souls looking for a home? 'For though the Body dies the Soul shall live for ever.' 'Summer suns are glowing'—Oh no! Not again Bion—'over land and sea. Happy light is flowing'—for you but not for me. 'The bells of hell go ting-a-ling-a-ling' for her but not for me. The Body lives for ever.

11

THE RAF were fed up and started the lorry with a jerk so as to throw the blasted bunch of officers out of the back. It was a short flight; I was decanted out at Croydon airport. Then Southbourne and the baby—a cheerful little mite and apparently glad to see me. My mother and father were anxious as if they expected me to be in a bad way. Would I consent to have the baby adopted? Of course there would be formalities . . . I was too outraged to understand that it was intended to be a serious question. Thick, slow-witted as ever, I undid the mass of ordnance towels I had been allowed to buy—and, crowning glory, zip fasteners! How Betty would have . . . she had mentioned how awkward it was never to be able to get zip fasteners for a number of jobs she would have to do—especially when the baby was born. When? That was *now.*

People were very helpful; someone said they knew of an arrangement that could temporarily provide the baby with all the care needed for the first year. "No", I said. I seemed unable to think of any other word to use.

I joined the suburban souls of sub-men and sub-women with sub-souls. I did not know who to be or what to be when death took my mate who was not a coward, and left me with a baby and £8000 to get on with. The £8000 we had saved out of my pay 'just in case.' In case what? I would have done better if I had had the sense to make the best of a bad job. In fact it seems now that it has always been the bad jobs, the hated jobs, the terrifying jobs that have made some sense of me.

The war, so they said, ended. Tub-thumping Montgomery, who fortunately knew how to thump other things besides tubs, broke out of the bridgehead at Rouen, trapped the big German forces sent to throw him out of France, and with the aid of his Air Force destroyed a considerable number of Wehrmacht. Later, the ability of the American forces to thump tubs made me aware that thumping tubs has a long history and great achievements to its credit: thumping one's own chest can produce a sound though the reverberations may be slight; the brave music of a distant drum has often attracted attention;

a boxer can attract much attention by thumping, in a drumlike manner, someone else's chest; combined with musical sounds such as singing it evokes widespread response. The response is lethal for some individuals. I could elicit agreement from Betty to going abroad in response to the call of duty—'I could not love thee dear so much, loved I not honour more.' What killed Betty and nearly killed her baby? Physical malformation? Incompetent obstetrics? Callous or indifferent authorities? Or the revelations of the hollow nature of the masculine drum that was being so loudly beaten by her husband's departure? Or was there something false about the psychiatric tones, the psychiatric pressure waves that were being set up? How would a sensitive conductor feel if God or Fate or the Devil condemned him to an eternity of eliciting a harmonious response from a tone-deaf, malicious, instrumentally armed orchestra?

We won the Second World War? The only part I noticed was that I was spending my resources of military gratuity, being the only psychiatrist I knew who ended in the same rank as he started; and I am proud to say that I at least allowed myself to recognize that one ended, as one started, by not existing. 'Man that is born of woman has very little time to live. He goes up like a top-gallant foresail and down like a small flying jib', as some poet has succinctly described it. I hope Betty enjoyed those brief years of fame that she had in fact achieved. Her baby—our baby—was now dependent on a woman who had given her mother such shelter as could be•afforded in smoky, blacked-out Slough, and now cared for her while her impecunious and unsuccessful father contemplated the rainbow-hued future.

I cannot remember being awarded a Victory Medal, but I am sure that a grateful establishment would have inflicted one on my completion of so many years of undetected nothingness, the ribbon designed in lavish colours of a nightmare of a 'morning after the night before'.

12

I HEARD of a cottage in Iver Heather—all the modern, British-style, conveniences—to be auctioned. With the best legal opinion from a very capable solicitor, who later came 'unstuck' by falling into the lawyer's booby trap or 'occupational neurosis', my bid of £8000 was successful. By curious chance I overheard a conversation in my Dorset Square Hotel between two well-informed and financially knowledgeable gentlemen who were talking in undisguised tones of mingled amusement and amazement about a fool who had just paid £8000 at auction for a mere workman's cottage. Could folly go further? And what were things coming to when that sort of fool could have £8000 to throw away? This story had an unpleasantly evocative quality. I listened; in fact I would have had to be deaf not to hear. My cottage was not in a particularly desirable neighbourhood either—poor train service and no buses worth talking about. Could that fool possibly be me? It could; it was.

In two particulars it was wrong: I did not have £8000 to throw about from lavish resources, and there *was* a bus service that I later had a good reason to talk about as one of those buses nearly killed me. Otherwise, I found on joining the conversation, the facts were correct and applied to me—a very close, if not exact fit.

I moved from Dorset Square to the cottage at Iver on the same day that the family looking after my baby moved in from Slough. The cottage was well built and adequate to shelter from rain. The garden included fine apple trees and ample ground for vegetables for the entire household. In conformity with the would-be prestige proper to a successful doctor, but not in conformity with the failure that bitter experience had taught me I was, I acquired a consulting room in a house in Harley Street. After a surprisingly short period I was amazed to find I had enough patients and such an acute shortage of cash that I had to work from nine to six on week-days, and nine to two on Saturday and Sunday. It was luxury and enough leisure for the acquisition of wisdom. I could not say I was a man learned enough to acquire wisdom; such thoughts I dismissed from my mind.

In the cottage garden there was a bush of wayfarer of which the leaves had turned deep red. I would not have remarked its presence but for the fact that the baby had forgotten me and expressed her displeasure at being held in the clumsy arms of a strange man. By chance her flailing limbs met the leaves of this plant and set them dancing. Fascinated by the sight, her cries ceased and her struggles changed to dancing in sympathy with the leaves. I was forgotten—and almost at once forgiven. In due course we moved on to other investigations.

I acquired a strongly built bicycle, said to be used by the police force and therefore adapted to a heavy load. With this was a carrier in which the baby could sit so that she had an uninterrupted view such as a pilot might get from his seat in an aircraft. I provided the motor force. Thus we would set out every Saturday to have tea in Denham village. It was not, gastronomically speaking, a remarkable tea but the ride there and home was an event that had a profound and deeply satisfying effect on me. I hoped it had a similarly profound effect on Parthenope.

Parthenope?

It was the name that Betty and I had decided should be the child's if it were a girl. Immediately after the event I wanted the name to be her mother's; then, that the name which had been born in the last agreed action of our life together should stand. 'Illo Vergilium me tempore dulcis alebat Parthenope . . .'[1] All that I had to do was to equal Virgil to fulfil any part of the contract—another certain failure, but *that* one I could not mind!

The week was not so satisfactory. Some problems were obvious: I had to have money to feed myself and the other inhabitants of the house. If enough patients wanted to see me I could be paid by them for . . . For what? The beauty of my physique? My knowledge of medicine? I had no assets in either respect even with the good fortune of having existed through two wars without being physically mutilated. Even my injured knee had been acquired trying to achieve athletic fame. Further debts that had been incurred did not obtrude into my awareness any more than they did, as appeared later, with the rest of the country.

Well, you've had a nice big war—two in fact—so now what about this little item? Excuse me, it's the Bill.

What? Do I have to pay for it too? You didn't mention that to me in August 1914.

[1] Virgil, Georgics Bk. IV. 'At that time I, Virgil, was being nourished by sweet Naples . . .'

Ah, but I did. Die for your country! Like that clever little doggie at Windsor.

Yes, but he didn't die. He went on wagging his tail.

Yes, but you have gone on living. All you have to do is to wag your little tail too!

I only have a vestigial tail—I can't wag that.

No, but you have a couple of nice cerebral hemispheres at the other end of your anatomy. Why don't you use them?

I though my parents and grandparents used them.

Sorry sir, they were too busy adoring their Maker.

Oh well, all right. Just put it on the bill. Two great wars and victories. I'll pay later.

Yes, certainly sir. In whose name shall I make it out? Your baby's? Or her children's children?

I couldn't think of all that and no one—

Oh come now; what about Oxford University?

—said I had to *use* my brain. And how do I *think* anyway? Especially with you interrupting the whole time.

Sorry sir. I'll just put it down to your daughter and her *offspring. She's too young to mind anyway.*

Here, half a minute—I didn't say that. He's disappeared without waiting for an answer. And it has quite spoiled my week-end. How can I wag my vestigial tail when I am made to think? Obviously—work at both ends, below and above the umbilicus, caudal *and* cranial.

13

I BECAME acutely aware of a sense of gratification when the bus stopped beneath a magnificent beech tree and I got off to be met by a small figure, now a toddler, doing her best to run to meet me. Her eyes were almost closed in the throes of concentration required for mobility and the equal necessity for concentration on where she was going. At last the perilous ten yards would be achieved and tiny arms strove to meet round my neck. A rapid change into week-end clothes, and then the cycle ride.

All this gratifying world now began to be invaded by thought. The calm fascination of picking, coring and slicing the excellent and plentiful Bramley apples preparatory to bottling them in a sulphur preparation for storage in an array of huge jars discarded by the sweetshop, became troubled by the doubts which flowed over the boundaries of my consulting room and the week's work and seeped into my private life and home. It was no longer private.

The invasion could not be repelled or contained. It is an invasion if one allows oneself to be aware of it; unfortunately it does not cease to be an invasion if one chooses to be, and succeeds in being, *unaware* of it. This should have been evident when the country had ceased to be aware of German aspirations to break out of the limitations thoughtfully provided by the 'victorious' allies in 1919. Had the allied powers not given the German authorities a plausible reason to feel enclosed, perhaps they would have had to realize that the compositions of Wagner, the lucubrations of Goethe, no more afforded adequate scope for expression of the Nazi violence. My present invasion of the realms of speculation about International Relations did not solve my resistance to the confinement of being satisfied with my home and professional life.

Rickman tentatively suggested that our war experience precluded the possibility of pursuing my analysis further. With this I agreed, for I had already considered the possibility of approaching Melanie Klein.

Melanie Klein, of whom I had heard and had had some chance of observing from a distance on one or two occasions, was a handsome, dignified and somewhat intimidating woman. My experience of association with women had not been encouraging or conducive to the growth of any belief in a successful outcome. However, I went to see her. I tried to indicate that I was worthy of her consideration, but she did not understand, or chose not to know—I don't know which—the enormous significance of the DSO. As I had not succeeded in believing that it was more than a cosmetic cover for my cowardice, the reality of which was never in the least doubt since I knew what it felt like to have *my* feelings, I thought that her ignorance might be reinforced by her disbelief in my masculine excellence. I had, in short, no evidence to support my application. She nevertheless agreed to accept me. How I was to pay my fees and read the psycho-analytic theories of Melanie Klein—I had looked at them and could not make head or tail of what I read—I had no idea.

My analysis pursued what I am inclined to think was a normal course: I retailed a variety of preoccupations; worries about the child, the household, financial anxieties—particularly how I was to find the money for such psycho-analytic fees *and* provide a home and care for the baby. Looking back on it I think my gifts as a sponger might have qualified me as a mendicant friar—unless of course that profession has some method of collecting from the friar such money as he collects or secretes. Mrs Klein remained unmoved and unmoving. I was very glad that she did, but that did not lead to the abandonment of my grievance. I suppose, reconsidering the matter, I expected to be supported in what I considered to be very moderate affluence. Why and on what grounds I thought the community required my continued existence is a puzzle, especially as I am now not likely to be eligible or desirable in any society—socially or militarily. Melanie Klein, however, was not easily led away from her awareness of a universe that is not subject to the needs and wishes of human beings, even when they came to her for analysis.

When I fell ill with jaundice and could not attend my sessions I still had to pay for them. As I had to pay for my illness by *not* being able to charge my patients fees for sessions *I* failed to keep, it did not take long to learn that illnesses or misfortunes are very expensive luxuries. Accordingly I turned up for one of my usual sessions without seeing any particular need to warn her that I was 'cured'—according to my doctor I was not—and that I was about to keep to my usual schedule. Mrs Klein was therefore taken by surprise and could not see me as she was fulfilling another engagement which she had made since she did not expect me. I returned to Iver.

I did not check my next account to see if she had charged me for a session which *she* had failed to keep. It may have been because I wished to preserve a grievance or because I had no expectations of obtaining redress; I do not know which.

I recovered, went back to work and my own analysis, swore 'never to do it again' and, as usual, invariably did again whatever it was I had sworn not to do. I was assiduous in my psycho-analytic sessions. When I was given an interpretation I used very occasionally to feel it was correct; more usually I thought it was nonsense but hardly worth arguing about since I did not regard the interpretation as much more than the expression of one of Mrs Klein's opinions that was unsupported by any evidence. The interpretations that I ignored or did not understand or made no response to, later seemed to have been correct. But I did not see why I regarded them as any more correct than I had thought they were when I refuted or ignored them. The most convincing were those that appeared to harmonize with what I knew, or what Mrs Klein said, about my personality. She tried to pass on to me her interpretations of the material of which her senses made her aware. But to become efficacious her methods were dependent on my receptivity. This is in no way different from any other form of human assistance—there must be someone or something willing to receive.

How banal is this conclusion! How obvious! And how perpetually that fact becomes clear and how frequently ignored. Yet a willing co-operation in teacher and taught is difficult to achieve when the participants are human. This banal observation seemed to be more than usually bitterly resisted when it was *I* who had to listen to what my senses told me, even with the assistance of Melanie Klein. But as time passed I became more reconciled to the fact that not even she could be a substitute for my own senses, interpretations of what my senses told me, and choice between contradictories. I did not become more amenable to her views but more aware of my disagreement. None the less there was something about that series of experiences with her that made me feel gratitude to her *and* a wish to be independent of the burden of time and expense of money and effort involved.

At last, after some years, we parted. She, I think, felt I still had a lot to learn from her but she agreed to the termination—partly no doubt through the realization that enough of WRB was enough.

I was, however, mistaken in thinking that we had seen the last of each other and that I was free to go. But I shall not anticipate that part of the story.

14

I REGAINED non-analytic consciousness to find I had a baby, a home, no wife but a simple, shrewd and helpful woman, and a father to whom I had offered my home since the death of my mother left him unwilling to live in a house haunted by memories of a dead partner who had shared a tempest-tossed and responsible career with him. I also acquired a practice without ever having come to a deliberate, conscious and voluntary decision to do so. I was paid, but since I had no money of my own beyond the remnants of a gratuity long since exhausted and a fund originally intended to support my wife and child in the event of my demise, the outlook seemed bleak. It was redeemed partly by the fact that my professional work was interesting, if not particularly valuable to the world in which I lived. Still, I hoped it might become so, as I felt no urge to devote myself to money-making.

I learned to stifle the wish, constantly awakened, that my infant's mother could see her and that we three together would go and have tea on Saturday afternoons. The facts were otherwise. Even the fact that I was not unhappy was something I resented. My father could not resist the temptation of making himself miserable by concentrating his mind on some improvement that should be made by himself, or myself, or both. I knew, and resented knowing, that he was right in so thinking. But what improvement?

A wife, of course. I did not need a psycho-analyst to tell me that. But *what* wife? I did not know of anyone, did not want to be reminded of Betty, did not want to be reminded of the girl who chose not to choose me.

That winter was very cold. The train in which I went from Uxbridge to Baker Street had automatic doors. These were opened at every station and left open so that passengers would have plenty of time in which to alight. Those who had not arrived at their destination found the time was adequate for losing any heat that they had acquired since awaking.

Harley Street in the Good Old Days was filled with real doctors, compassionate, highly qualified technicians. I could not be one of those as I had largely wasted my chance of becoming even technically proficient. But I could assume a plausible representation of one: the address on my headed notepaper, a gold medal for surgery that I had acquired in much the same incomprehensible way as I had won first prize for making a sandcastle at Hastings. After all, if your prize causes you to win a prize why not collect it? So, there it was—a Harley Street Specialist.

In the mean time patients came and paid. My fees, though small, were wealth to me and I could even afford—financially—meals that were bad for my health. So I could escape from the pains of indigence into the pleasures of gluttony.

Yet now I felt as never before; numbed and insensitive. That something was wrong, must be wrong, was brought home to me one week-end when I was sitting on the lawn near the house and the baby was crawling near a flower bed on the opposite side of the lawn. She began to call out to me; she wanted me to come to her.

I remained sitting. She now made to crawl towards me. But she called to me as if expecting me to come to fetch her.

I remained sitting.

She continued to crawl and now her calls became distressful.

I remained sitting.

I watched her continue on the painful journey across the vast expanse, as it must have appeared to her, that separated her from her Daddy.

I remained sitting but felt bitter, angry, resentful. Why did she do this to me? Not quite audible was the question, "Why do you do this to her?"

The nurse could not stand it and got up to fetch her. "No," I said, "let her crawl. It won't do her any harm." We watched the child crawl painfully. She was weeping bitterly now but sticking stoutly to her attempt to cover the distance.

I felt as if I were gripped in a vice. No. I would *not* go. At last the nurse, having glanced at me with astonishment, got up ignoring my prohibition, and fetched her. The spell snapped. I was released. The baby had stopped weeping and was being comforted by maternal arms. But I, I had lost my child.

I hope there is no future life.

I had begged Betty to agree to have a baby: her agreement to do so had cost her her life.

I had vowed to look after the child. It was not a promise to Betty; it was an unexpected vow to myself. It was a shock, a searing shock, to find such depth of cruelty in myself. I have since often recalled Shakespeare's words: 'Nymph, in thy orisons be all my sins remembered'.[1]

[1] *Hamlet*, III. i.

THE OTHER SIDE OF GENIUS

I

Letters
To
Francesca

1951

The Homestead, Iver Heath

March 22

Francesca dear,

This does not seem to be a very sensible time in the morning to start writing you a letter but then I feel I cannot wait till tomorrow. Besides this is not *really* a letter but just a note and tomorrow I shall write a letter.

I walked back with a great wind blowing hazy clouds across a moon which was never visible but made all the trees stand out a deep grey against the silvery meadows and water. And all the time I could see you, and still see you, looking more ravishingly beautiful, as you did all the evening when I was with you, than any one could believe possible. You were kind to be like that.

And here I shall have to stop for my thoughts will not flow freely when I feel that all I would say cannot be written—or certainly not when I keep thinking of mundane things such as whether I shall be in time to catch a morning post with this, or even whether there is a morning post on a Good Friday.

So, goodbye dear Francesca till tomorrow when I shall be writing you a letter. Remember me, please, to your Mother and give her my best Easter wishes.

Dear Francesca, bless you.

With love from

Wilfred

March 23

Francesca dear,

. . . My mind is so filled with last night and next Tuesday that I don't find I concentrate very well on the present. Not that today has been exactly the sort of day that insists on being noticed; the morning was pleasant enough but since then it has come down in buckets. I am rather lucky because I love weather—all sorts of weather. I think there is a lot to be said for being born, as I was, in India. To me, rain was of course the great event, the monsoon, and I can even now, though I left India when I was eight, recapture the thrill of the smell of parched land rain-soaked—something of an effort these last two months . . .

Saturday morning. I felt so tired that I dropped off to sleep thinking I would wake half an hour later and write some more. Instead, though it was only 10.30 when I went to sleep, I found when I awoke it was ten this morning. This always happens when holiday breaks come. I don't remember that I must be tired, because I don't usually feel tired, discover I can do no work, and then have a deep sleep and feel better. I am now trying to write this, alone in the house with Parthenope, to a continuous stream of interruptions from P. who wants to know everything from, What shall I do now? to, How do you spell oranges? I think one should learn to develop a split mind for doing two things at once and talking about another one, all at the same time.

I have just seen a notice in the paper about 'The Consul'[1] from Alan Dent in which he is most urgent that everyone should see it. It has only a week to go and I wondered if it was so good that you would care to see it again and would have the time to come with me if I could get seats. I could ring up for seats on Tuesday, I expect, because I doubt whether Alan Dent's notice will have the effect of filling it up.

It looks a pretty gusty sort of day for the boat race. I shall watch it on television (or rather I shall have my eyes firmly fixed on the launches in the vague but unlikely hope that I shall see you) but I don't think there is any doubt that Cambridge will walk away with it. If it blows clear, and there seems some sign of it, you may have a very enjoyable time; there is something very fascinating to me about the preliminary excitements. Even when I was taking part I rather used to enjoy 'having the needle'.

Parthenope has stopped asking questions and is now telling herself fairy stories, "so you can't hear", and the silence is almost as devastating as the interruptions . . .

March 24

Francesca dear,

. . . We duly saw Oxford sink on the television and I hoped you weren't there. Even a launch would have been an uncomfortable experience on such a day, not to mention the disappointment of 'no race'. It is astonishing how clear the television pictures are, even expressions are visible.

[1] The opera by Giancarlo Menotti.

It is a marvellous moonlit night with the wind sighing gently in the pine trees. There is a line of Flecker's which goes:

For pines are gossip pines the wide world through.[1]

It has always stuck in my mind since I first came across it when I was at Oxford. Arthur Bryant[2] and I used to learn quite a lot of verse when we were up. But I think I learnt most during the first world war. My biggest feat was in 1918 I think when our battalion had no tanks left and I and a dozen of my men had to fill a gap in the line with our machine guns. Our last night before relief I was with a colonel of the Royal Scots and it became clear as we were talking that a German night attack was starting. As everything that could be done had been done he said, Let's talk about something decent. Have you read the de Coverly essays? I told him I had, so we talked about Sir Roger de Coverly and Will Wimple and the rest while the Boche in his little way shelled our waterlogged line of shell-holes and earthworks to bits. The colonel got killed a little later, and I, still having nothing to do, learned off 'L'Allegro' and 'Il Pensoroso' from a Golden Treasury I had with me. As it turned out we were only on the flank of the attack and were relieved a little before dawn. I don't think I remember much of either now though funnily enough I can still repeat a good deal of Virgil that I learnt at, though not 'in', school. I hated Latin lessons but used to like the sound of Virgil so I used to learn bits. We never 'did' the Georgics which I think the best of the lot.

Easter Sunday. I want to add more to this before I go to catch the Sunday post which goes at tea-time. It is still a lovely afternoon and has all the promise of Spring about it. Many birds are singing and for the first time I have seen in this garden what I think was probably the lesser spotted woodpecker; the green woodpecker that makes the lovely laughing call is quite common and often lands on the lawn, despite our cat.

I shall try this afternoon to finish off corrections of a first draft I have of a contribution[3] to a book edited by Roger Money-Kyrle.[4] The sky has become rather grey so I daresay there will be more rain tonight. Poor bank holiday people!—they have had a wretched Easter so far . . .

Dear Francesca, goodbye: I did not know four days could ever pass so slowly.

[1] James Elroy Flecker, 'Brumana'.
[2] Sir Arthur Bryant, the historian.
[3] 'Language and the Schizophrenic'.
[4] *New Directions in Psycho-analysis*, Tavistock Publications Ltd., 1955.

March 26

Francesca dear,
There does not seem the least chance that I shall be able to write a letter any more than I can do anything else but I want to send something by post before it goes. I cannot correct my draft or do anything sensible . . .

I took Parthenope for a walk this morning in a slight drizzle of rain. Despite the fact that this is nothing but a country slum, the worst kind of slum of all I think, it was very pleasant as it was warm and the birds were singing. But the hedgerows are surprisingly backward. I usually reckon on a green blush in the hedges by Lady Day[1] but although it has not been cold there is nothing. It looks almost as if they did not like the rain.

I stop every now and then to think about tomorrow and indeed there is nothing else whatever in my head and I can't just go on writing to you saying, I wonder if you will have a blue bow in your hair, or the yellow one, or the mauve one (if 'bow' is the right term) and whether you will have one at all and—this you will think strange—what you really look like. I almost have to try to remember by the photographs you showed me! And I am frightened I shall just be struck dumb like a blithering idiot; even now it makes me catch my breath when I see you in my mind's eye.

I have taken so long over this worthless epistle that I must now seal it up and take it to the post. Be patient with me dear Francesca.

March 28

Francesca my darling,
This is only a note to say I love you. What a pity it would be so dull if I only filled the page up with those three words because they are the only ones that seem to go through my head. How wonderful to be John Donne and able to write you 'The Extasy'. How enviable to pour out 'La ci darem' la mano' instead of remaining chained in inarticulateness.

Well, there it is; so I shall have to say instead that I had a long wait at Baker Street, did not bother waiting, perhaps fruitlessly, for a taxi at Uxbridge, and so walked home without being smothered in rain or swallowed up in a snow drift. Parthenope was crying out just as I came in, presumably with a nightmare. How people can think of childhood as 'happy' I do not know. A horrible bogey-ridden, demon-haunted time it was to me and then one has not the fortitude, or callosities perhaps, with which to deal with it.

[1] March 25.

I am finding it very difficult even to take any notice of the daily life around me but look forward yearningly to our next meeting. I am going on writing this in the morning as my eyes were too heavy with sleep last night. It takes me an enormous time to write these letters because I stop at every other word to think about you, or I should say to dream about you.

On second thoughts I don't think I want to be Donne or Mozart (perhaps in the event it is just as well). I don't think even they can have found it very satisfactory: really all I want is to be able to be with you. I feel quite worried that I can think of nothing else because I do not want to become a terrible bore. I am very glad you don't want to be Vicereine: not only because it would mean having to reconquer India. Even in my insignificant life there are so many demands on my time that I feel I have no private life and you must have so many friends who will certainly not let you go, as well as your work, that I shall have to learn how to remain cool, calm and collected in face of great frustration.

Francesca my darling love I worship and adore you. These are the words that you must understand are disguised in the volume of poems I gave you last night.[1] People can think it is just a date. I hope my life, our life, my life that now belongs to you, will be of such a kind that the whole world around us, but more particularly you yourself, will know that they must be true. Francesca darling, does this sound very solemn—too solemn? I feel it all. I don't feel a bit like what I expected to feel and yet I thought I knew . . .

March 29

Francesca, my darling love,
To-night I had the good luck to get a lift in a taxi that was just moving off with a fare to Iver Heath so I had no wait at all and no walk through a dismal drizzle of rain. What a wonderful evening it has been. 'The Consul' was an immensely moving experience and what added to the depth of my happiness was the knowledge that but for you I would not have had it. Your presence pours a soft radiance of joy over my life . . .

I was just settling down to go on with this after lunch when Ken Rice phoned through. I find it hard to say why I felt so tongue-tied when he spoke to me but I just suddenly felt, when I knew you had told him, that what he was saying was about something so terribly important in my life that I could hardly keep a tremble out of my

[1] The complete poems of Robert Frost.

voice any more than I could keep it out of my hands as I held a wobbling receiver to my ear. Similarly I feel very nervous about ringing anyone up myself although I have now told Mary Hall, the wife of a very old friend of mine who is the medical officer for Bucks; I was best man at his wedding before the last war.

Everything seems to have gone out of my mind but the thought of seeing you again tomorrow. In my heart I hear the proud love of Handel's music to—

Where'er you walk cool gales shall fan the glade;
Trees, where you sit, shall crowd into a shade;
Where'er you tread the blushing flowers shall rise,
And all things flourish where'er you turn your eyes.

To me it means one thing and one thing only, for now and for ever, my darling Francesca.

It has been a lovely day, cold but sunny and clear with maybe a promise of something good for tomorrow.

I have just discovered that it is nearly time for the last post so I had better seal this up and post it. My letters to you have no ending—no sooner have I posted one that I start writing my next one. But for the present I shall say goodbye. My darling sweetheart Francesca I love you; I love you.

April 1

Francesca darling,

It is very doubtful if I shall manage to write anything at all as I have by my side Parthenope painting, sworn to vows of silence, absolute and eternal, till released by me. But the Trappist vows are, I find, not absolute but relative when it comes to practice, so do not be surprised if this letter is disjointed and has a harrassed and worried tone. I can't stop writing even for a moment as it is the signal for an outburst of requests, questions and so on. The silences are of much the same duration as the 'bright intervals' we hear about these days.

I woke up at what I thought was five minutes to nine but only to discover, on closer inspection, that it was a quarter to eleven, having slept like a log from the moment I dropped my head on the pillow. Pretty late it is true. I tried to ring up Sutherland before lunch but found he was out—at least the phone remained unanswered. But I did get Trist, complaining bitterly of overwork, who was very pleased at the news.

Bless you my dearest sweetheart for all you are. How much you mean to me I cannot say: I want to feel that I shall be able to go on trying to find ways of saying it through the years.

I wonder if I shall be able to get on the track of a ring at all tomorrow. I want to find a ring which does not show all its secrets to the stranger. It would be wonderful if we could find one with a deep richness that made you feel it had a fire glowing within it to warm your heart and make you feel: The man that gave me this loves me for myself alone and forever.

Parthenope's silence has been *a tour de force* but if you are at the receiving end of it it is not conducive to concentration. The actual moments when she is not talking are even worse than the questions, it is so painful to see the agonized efforts required to refuse utterance to the latest inspiration.

My love dear.

April 1

My darling love,

A most exhausting day; I have been compelled to be made an April Fool so often by my enthusiastic Parthenope that I am quite worn out. The stimulation of surprise, indignation and mortification demands histrionic powers that are quite beyond me without the exercise of great effort.

Your remark that you did not know what relatives I have has made me think I should devote this letter to letting you know about the awful sort of family that you are now about to become a member of—the Bions. The first and fundamental thing to realize is that they are all, as far as I am aware without exception, completely cracked. This is the more difficult because they possess a sort of cunning that has kept them out of the looney bin. I haven't been able to keep track of them all so I shall concentrate on the most important members

First of all there was a grandfather Robert Bion who was some sort of missionary in India. I don't know anything about him although there is a pamphlet knocking around somewhere proving that he was a 'fine man'. He had three, or maybe four, sons, one of which I knew as Uncle Bertie who married someone called Irene, worked in the Indian railways, once gave me a tip, and disappeared, for ever as far as I know, from my young life. There were then three brothers: the eldest my Uncle Walter, then my Uncle Rupert and last my father. All are now dead. To prove they were quite mad they married three sisters of a family called Kemp—probably missionary or 'off' missionary in the sense that builders and decorators talk about 'off' white when they mean cream coloured. The eldest married my Uncle Walter. She was my Aunt Helen who was as mad as her husband. Then came my Aunt Alice who married my Uncle Rupert, and last my mother who was called Rhoda. All had children. I shall take them in turn starting at the eldest, my Uncle Walter and Aunt Helen.

Oh, I had forgotten: there was another uncle and aunt but I don't think I ever saw them and have forgotten their names; missionaries, but I always had some contact with their children, Marguerite, Herbert and Arnold. The reason I have forgotten them is that I was very fond of them and they were all quite sane and therefore only resembled Bions because they had the same name. To me they were always something special as you shall hear when I come to them if your patience has taken you so far.

Darling Francesca: I have just been in a day dream again thinking with longing of your dear presence. I find that quite trivial moments seem fixed deep in my heart; for some reason moments such as one when, after I went to look for a taxi when we came out of Kettner's, I looked back and saw you standing waiting in the distance under the theatre. There seems no reason why one particular moment like that should be so clear to my sight but so it is. And I long for the time, though I grudge it too, when I shall be able to bring my friends to you to meet you. I feel so proud of you, my true and only love, that I want to have people see you while I stand by and say, There! Look! Aren't I a fine fellow to have such great happiness? Have you ever seen such a beautiful woman as my Francesca? my darling Francesca?

Your letter came this morning together with one from Jaques congratulating me. I had to put it in my pocket and keep it for a long time before reading it so that I could keep saying to myself, I have a letter from Francesca, from my darling.

It's no good trying to go on with the family history now and in any case it is time I was getting ready to go up to Town. I am very anxious to find a ring which you will be very fond of even if we have to wait a little while to find one which is just what you would want to have. I cannot hope to find one that will satisfy me, that I know, but I think if you are particular about it and don't let yourself be hurried into something that does not feel quite right I shall learn to love it because it is yours.

And now my dear love I shall have to stop. With all my love Francesca my darling.

Till I see you sweetheart, goodbye.

[Undated]

Francesca my darling,

I have just got back from the group so I shall try to dash off a short note to you. I found the discussion interesting and I am pleased to say that although I found myself handicapped by my lack of reading which is always my weak point I made up for by my ability not to lose sight of the wood for the trees. And again I think my contribution licked the discussion into shape and gave it a meaning and coherence which it had not before. There is great pleasure to be had in a group which so quickly grasps one's point and seems so ready to acknowledge the value of the contribution. Very egotistical perhaps but I confess that it pleases me.

I have just remembered that I shall be free on Saturday morning as I need not go up to Town till late—Melanie is off work. It will probably be a good thing if I put in some work here arranging for the house to be sold or at least tidied ready for sale.

My darling you looked quite breath-takingly lovely today; even now I feel the thrill as I see you in my mind's eye. How I long to have you in my arms. And then I think how much I just want to sit and watch you, my dear sweetheart. Once I start thinking like this it is goodbye to all letter writing. I go into a daze of happiness and there is no more question of 'dashing' off a note to you . . .

Now my dearest I will stop. I shall try to go off to sleep. All my love to you my darling.

April 6

Francesca, my darling,

It was kind of you to give me such a lovely scarf; I say 'lovely scarf' but I am really very well aware that to me the really exciting thing is that it comes to me from my darling. As for the note, I was torn between my desire to store it up and save it for carefully reading every word, and my desire to tear it open and read it at once. I think I behaved very well don't you? Quite nonchalent and calm and collected all through tea-time and all the way back to Harley Street. Then I *had* to open the main envelope but I kept the letter burning in my pocket till the interval between the first patient and the next. Now wasn't that an admirable display of phlegm? My dear, what an adorable postscript! I don't know how I got from Harley Street to Iver without any awareness of the intervening stages. One of these days someone who knows me will see me in the train, and then whatever will they think? Sweetheart, it would not surprise me at all if they were to think I must be in love.

Darling Francesca, I can hardly write a letter. I need hours to think about the scarf; then I find I need hours to think about the letter; I hardly have time to think about either when I realize I must have a long, long time to think over carefully and slowly every detail of your astonishing loveliness as you sat at tea. The scarf about your shoulders, your ear-rings, my heart beats faster as I see you again as I write. In my heart I feel that *there* is a present such as no one in the world but you my darling could give me, a present that fills me with such deep joy that it is almost pain. I never believed that the Tavi[1] could be a beautiful place to me but 'where'er you tread the blushing flow'rs shall rise' . . .

. . . I feel the one thing that can make all things possible already exists, and that is that between you and me there is already an enduring love that cannot be easily shaken even in this uncertain and painful world. I am more thankful than I can say that something gave me the courage to know that when I found that you had become the first person in my heart, that was the right and proper foundation without which one would build in vain, no matter what one tried to do. In my heart today I knew when I put your portrait over the mantlepiece in Harley Street that it meant what I deeply felt. Something seemed to whisper to me, sharp and clear, That is right, that is as it should be; do not be afraid. Darling Francesca, without you I am nothing.

'Sorrow follows folly as the berries grow on holly and—
Oh! 'tis folly—to be afraid of love.'

Francesca darling, you are a miracle that has happened to me, a miracle that I do not understand or ever want to understand. Enough for me that it has happened.

It is now Saturday evening and as usual I have been sitting in front of the paper unable to go on because as soon as I think of you I become lost in a day dream of seeing you again. I must tell you of the tragedy of the Second Cup of Tea at tea-time yesterday. I became aware of it with a flash of annoyance just as I got up to fetch my second cup and realized, when it was too late, that all the time I was away fetching it I should not be with you. The tragedy arose because, ever since I had first seen you at the Tavi, I had taken to paying for more than one cup of tea, although I didn't want it, because it gave me an excuse not only to hang on longer over my tea and therefore see you as much as possible, but also a double chance of being at the tea urn, perhaps at the same time as you were. So, automatically I

[1] The Tavistock Clinic and The Tavistock Institute of Human Relations, then in Beaumont Street.

carried out my usual technique without thinking, and found of course that I had lost precious moments out of what was already a very small supply.

. . . When I ring you up again soon, happy thought, though I know I shall be tantalized almost beyond endurance, I shall ask you if you think I should fix up the Halls for tomorrow tea-time. Stevie Hall is a very old friend of mine. He was just at school with me though much junior and I didn't know him except as a name. But we have always kept up a contact ever since; after the first war, I became engaged to his sister for a short time though I completely lost all contact with her. It is hard to be objective about someone you like, especially if he likes you sufficiently to ask you to be his best man at his wedding. I think of him as one of these alert lively people, always very successful at school—he became Head Prefect before he left. He has got to the top, or thereabouts, of his particular tree; reads a lot, meets interesting people and plans to send his boys to Eton which is a school I admire but would in no circumstances be my choice even in the unlikely event of my being able to afford such a place. They seem to me to let far too many boys go hang and after all they are only children and need care.

Last night I told another of my old friends. He is George Mitchell and dates from my arrival at Oxford as an undergraduate after the first war. George is a batchelor and looks it. We meet perhaps once a year and then not at all for some years. He is bald-headed, thin, dyspeptic-looking, careworn, filled with a kind of canny realism that he partly inherited and partly acquired at Rugby. You would be right in supposing he looks a decrepit old city magnate; but he was born looking like that, of that I am convinced. Anyhow he was exactly like that at Oxford. He and I used to go and argue philosophy with Paton, now professor of Philosophy at Glasgow University, then a don at Queen's which was the seat of learning that George and I graced with our presences. His brains rather intimidated me then, but I have since grown to think I have more—I mean I began to think so even before the last week; I don't count *since* our engagement because, as you know, I have now become quite convinced I must be a *very* remarkable person. He busies himself in good works—Leader of the Opposition in the L.C.C., something-or-other running University College Hospital (where I trained). He was on the Stock Exchange but gave it up as he didn't like money-making. He must in fact be very well off I imagine, as he occasionally buys a good picture; I think he gives shrewd and good business advice to people who would otherwise not be able to get it. The cultured Rugbeian is a nice man to meet but there are some rough ones—many I daresay if one knew those that had not gone on to a university.

Darling Love, I have sat in front of this sheet blankly for half an hour since I wrote the previous lines simply thinking how wonderful it felt when you said you would ring me up tomorrow morning before you left to come here. It is like the P.S. and P.P.S. to your letter. I think it utterly wonderful that you do that for me. She does it for *me*, I say to myself, trying to grasp it.

Dear Darling Francesca: I have taken so long over this that I *must* stop or I shall not have time to sleep. I long for you.

Dear love, goodnight.

April 10

Francesca my darling,

Even though it is so late I must just send you this tiny note. Sweetheart it was lovely to hear your dear voice: I worked quite well all day I think, and really quite enjoyed meeting Ken largely because he knew without my saying anything how deeply I felt about you and what a tremendous thing it was for me that such a beautiful woman loved me; yet when I found I could not get through to you I suddenly realized how badly I was missing you and how much strain it meant. I suddenly felt tired out and from that time on the hands of the clock simply crawled. I felt I must get home to the telephone, that I could hardly endure another moment without the sound of your sweet voice. And yet I managed to read some Fowler[1] on the way back, sensibly too, so it must be a good sort of agony. Dear Sweetheart, my work is coming alive; the dull numb mechanical routine into which I have fallen is bursting wide open and it is all you my darling, my darling Francesca . . .

April 11

Francesca my darling,

Another good-night note from me which I expect will be a good-morning note to you. We had quite a good meeting although I felt a little too much in the clouds to take a proper part in it. There is something very satisfactory about working in a small group of five people all of whom have a keen intelligence and a good grasp of the subject. But they started by each congratulating me very warmly on our engagement and if anything was needed to send my mind chasing off to the place where my heart now rests, that provided it. I really must start reading some psycho-analysis soon or people will

[1] *Modern English Usage.*

think you have made a *very* queer choice. Dr Heimann, who is the best in the group by far, is very insistent that we live in St. John's Wood —I knew she would be. She is a very warm-hearted woman.

Darling! Monday is all right: the patient I was to see cannot come till May so a great cloud is lifted from my heart. Can you keep Monday evening at 7.30 free?

Even the short time tonight was a great solace to me. My sweetheart you had put in day's work and I really did not care hope to see you although I expect, after my experience yesterday, that I should have felt dreadful if I had had to go right through till tomorrow without a sight of you. Dear Francesca—how much you mean to me.

I felt so happy when you spoke of a nursery. The mere thought of *our* children is inexpressibly sweet to me. You have given Parthenope back to me and made me feel what it is like to have a child. You cannot think how terrible it has been to feel all the time that every day she was becoming more lost to me till at times she hardly seemed my child at all. I know now, and rejoice in knowing, that miraculous as it seems to me that it should be so, yet my love matters to you. And deeply as I feel this I yet feel infinitely happy to think that you may know a still deeper love than this and that is the love for your own child.

Darling Francesca; may you have a very happy week-end. You will be in my heart always, a glow of happiness that is my darling Love.

April 12

Francesca, my darling,

I have just been thinking of the house,[1] having read the detailed description on the way home. I wonder if you think it will need a lot of painting or if you think that there is enough of it 'liveable in' to do some of the work ourselves when we are in. I have both a petrol driven pump and sprays that will do whitewashing very efficiently and fast, and an electrical paint gun. We could use these ourselves if you felt inclined to make a hobby of decorating, say one room to suit our own tastes. . . But I must not go on like this or I shall have imagined a totally impractical dream house which will make me feel quite dissatisfied with any real house we are likely to meet.

Darling, your choice of ring[2] seems to me to become more and more right; it looks lovely on your hand; you must be able to do something even to diamonds . . .

[1] Redcourt.
[2] A French ring, dated 1740.

April 13

My darling,

As usual I was too overwhelmed at tea-time to be able to say anything then or afterwards. It was a great comfort and pleasure to me to have your letter. I am sorry I could only give you my tiny scrap. Actually I had felt exactly the same—that you and I ought to see the house together, but I was torn by the thought that you were having a very hard rush of work and were already much too tired, so I thought before suggesting it I would wait till I saw you today.

I have had some nice letters: indeed one of the things that has touched me has been the amount of affection and good will there is to us. Needless to say those who know you have no doubt at all that I am a very lucky man, a glimpse of the obvious, but how good it is to hear you praised and feel the affection and pride in which you my darling are held. My solicitor wrote a very pleasant letter. John Bowlby wrote very kindly and Sutherland, whom I rang up to-night and who is only just back from holiday, said that everyone in the Tavi is delighted and he sounded as if this were no conventional phrase. He also said that all the women in the Tavi that know you say how much they like you. John Rickman wrote congratulating me—I don't think you know him though. Then I got a very charming letter from Colonel Alex—the brother of the Field Marshal and my late CO—sending us both good wishes from himself and his wife. I am very fond of Alex: I always got on with him very well indeed. He wanted to know when the wedding is . . .

And—what are we going to do about the wedding? It sounds to me as if we shall have to put if off till we have saved enough money to hire the Albert Hall or Olympia for a reception!

I asked a taxi man today and he told me that from Victoria to Harley Street would take 10 minutes at most in the morning, as the streets are clear, and would cost 2/– or 3/–, so that is obviously the answer. I am hoping this may mean that I could leave home (home!) at about 8.50 instead of 8.15 and that will make a big difference to me over the week. But I notice already that whereas before (Before Francesca) even one late night a week left me tired out by the week-end, now tonight I feel as fresh as paint. I feel quite troubled and guilty at all the work you have been doing. It is wonderful to me that despite the tiredness you feel, you look so wonderful. I like to hear about your "horrible conceit"; my only comment would be to quote the Frenchman's remark about Curzon—"immense orgeuil—justifié".

Darling I must stop although I feel I have not said a tenth of what I want to write. Goodnight, dear heart.

April 17

Francesca, my darling,
The sound of your voice has made me feel so much better that I must just write this little note. Already I feel impatient for tea-time. You cannot imagine how good I feel when you say you will fetch me a cup of tea. Darling, I love your doing things for me: I am just not used to it, that's all. I look at you and I can hardly believe my eyes; then my heart tells me it is really true.

Dearest, I *am* looking forward to Mrs Riviere's party. She is a somewhat formidable woman, but a well-wisher of mine and I anticipate feeling a very proud man when I appear in 'public' with you. I have a feeling that the evening will end with some more people thinking I have 'very good taste'. I shall try not to go round saying to people, "Aren't I *clever*!" but I expect I shall *look* like it whatever I do.

I've spent so long about this I must stop. Goodnight my darling: goodnight Francesca my dear love.
P.S. There are some kisses at the bottom right hand corner. They are rather crowded together.

April 21

Dearest,
I am waiting for the telephone to ring and for the sound of your dear voice. So you must not expect a letter from me; it is just not possible in these circumstances: I shall fall back on a dreary recital of the history of the Bion family in order to kill time and provide me with a soporific. Indeed it may serve a useful purpose by acting as a soporific for you too. To begin then I shall introduce you to the senior branch—the Walter Bions.

My Aunt Helen was a formidable woman, by nature kind but shrill and embittered by being married to my Uncle Walter. She had I think natural ability and must have been a very beautiful girl as she was handsome to the end. My Uncle Walter was the eldest of the Bion brothers and was described as a saintly and learned man reported to be able to read the New Testament in Greek. Actually he was a horrid little man who was happily as incompetent in his meanness as he was in his work. His incompetence at his work led my Aunt Helen to call him unworldly and from that it was but a short step to canonization as a saint. His temper was made no better by the manifest superiority of his two younger brothers, Uncle Rupert and my father, who were in their respective spheres brilliant and, it goes without saying when talking of Bions, impossible. Uncle Walter ultimately got a job in the Meteorological Department of the Indian government. In spite of the fact that for nine months of the year the sun beats down on the entire peninsula with pitiless heat, and the heavens open for the remaining three to drench the land with rain; in spite of the fact that the department refused resolutely to give my uncle any promotion whatsoever; so powerful was the effect of his mere presence on the pay-roll of the department that the predictions of the meteorological office were suffused with the glow of his incompetence and were hailed as masterpieces of comic mis-statement until he was forcibly retired to live in Upper Norwood where he devoted his energies, if such a word can be applied to a moribund amoeba, in equal proportions to church-going and the dissemination of a sort of mischievous religiosity through his household. The household consisted of my poor aunt, my shrewish cousin Beryl, now happily lost to sight, and a mongrel dog which suffered from delusions of persecution. The dog and I led to a family row, thuswise: my father and mother and I were visiting them for tea. Quite forgetting the appalling consequences that were almost certain to follow any display of bonhomie in such a household, I waved my hat cheerily at the dog. It immediately set up such an uproar of barking, snapping, foaming at the mouth and so forth that my uncle rushed out saying he would not have me ill-treating the dog. My father, hearing the racket, rushed out in his turn and, thinking I had been bitten by my Uncle Walter, became extremely angry with my uncle. Aunt Helen stood palefaced and erect unable to speak. My mother then appeared but by this time the scene was of such indescribable confusion—Uncle squeaking, Dad thundering maledictions, dog barking madly and self trying to find a hat peg—that she could make nothing of it. We had a very frigid tea, which was not unwelcome as it was an exceedingly hot day, and the two families did not speak to each other for a year or more.

My cousin Beryl was known, even from early childhood in India, as a horrible little sneak and was detested by her brothers Cyril and Melvin. Aunt Helen, who believed all her children to be extremely gifted, insisted she could sing. So every morning before breakfast she could be heard, in a thin quavering voice, singing very flat a song called, I believe, The Mountains of Marne. It used to bring tears to my aunt's eyes but she must have had some glimmering of the truth somewhere because she never unleashed Beryl to sing at anyone; always only 'practising' at the crack of dawn.

I liked my aunt. She used—I should say that all this was when I was 21 years old—to tell me ecstatically about India. The beauty of the birds particularly entranced her. "They have", she used to say, waving a languid hand as she sought for the *mot juste,* "such *glorious* foliage." "Plumage, Auntie", I would correct in my pedantic way. "Wilfred", she would reply in half mock anger, "don't put me out. You know very well what I mean." "Yes, Auntie", I would reply submissively, "I do; you mean plumage." My uncle would sit with furrowed brow reading an illiterate religious rag called 'The Life of Faith'. As far as I know he never read anything else not even the New Testament 'in original Greek'.

Poor Uncle Walter; right at the end when he was eighty odd he had a temporary phase of sanity and, realizing that he had wasted his life, became extremely cross with everyone and everything, so they shut him up in a looney bin. I always thought it very hard lines as it was really the only time in his life when I heard him say a sensible thing.

His eldest son Cyril, mad as a hatter like the rest of us, taught himself how to paint, but just had enough horse sense to marry, to the family disgrace, a very nice girl who was a shop assistant somewhere or other. She had the sense to make him get a schoolmastering job in Ireland where of course no one would notice anything peculiar, and there, as far as I know, he is still at large.

Melvin was a great hero of mine when I was six. He became an engineer, married and lived dully ever after.

I had nearly bored myself to sleep when . . . the telephone bell rang. So I cannot possibly return to this dreary subject again. My darling, how sweet it is to hear your voice. I feel very excited about the house, very excited indeed. And very guilty to think of all the work you have been doing while I sit about gazing into space gaping like a goldfish wondering how to pass the time till I see you again.

It is no good: I can't go on. I just see your dear face and dream of you, longing to see you and thinking how wonderful it would be to see you the mistress of the house. Darling I hope it will be as happy a one as you deserve and I can't say more than that.

After a long pause I have realized that unless I pull myself together and write some family history I shall never get to sleep. So I will end my account of the Walter Bions by two more pieces of information. Besides the paranoid mongrel there was a cat. This creature, which I had almost forgotten, was, unlike the dog, extremely depressed. There is nothing more to say about it; it was just extremely depressed.

My cousin Cyril used occasionally to visit them from Ireland. They all hated each other in a most malignant, noisy, and monotonous way until one day Cyril galvanized the whole party into stupefaction by maintaining—he still does I think—that Uncle Walter was not his father.

The effect of this on my uncle was bad enough but nothing at all compared with its effect on my poor aunt who instantaneously realized, since apparently he still considered her his mother, that the physiological implications of this, if translated into sociological or, still worse, theological terms, invited very sinister interpretations of her morality however flattering they might be to her charms.

Darling, it's no use trying to write more of this but I think I have written quite enough to send *you* to sleep if not myself. My mind and heart are all yours. I feel that we are on the start of a fine adventure and though I am filled with joy I think it a most solemn and happy thing. I know there will be plenty of difficulties to overcome but with you I feel I can face them with real happiness. We shall not be well-off, but I see so many who are not a ha'porth happier for it that I am full of hope that your home will be a happy one.

It is very late my darling so I shall say good-night. Dearest I love you.

With many, many kisses.

April 23

Francesca my darling,

I cannot promise more than a note as I am anxious not to stay up too late but this will be to send you my love. It was good to see you for a short time to-day and good to hear your voice on the phone. But I think we will have to get used to the frustration that both of us must feel just now—not an easy thing for either of us. If these feelings did not exist, disagreeable as they are, one would really wonder why they did not.

I am already looking forward to next Saturday; it will be our first appearance together and though it will be a small gathering I think it will be fun. There is something exciting about learning to act as a team.

Monday is always something of a strain for me. I find I have not got into the weekly rush and nearly always take far too long about dressing and such like, and so start off by being nearly late. And then it is a very full day so I am glad to see the end of it. Nevertheless in spite of the appearances I think I am doing good work with my patients even if I do not make any progress with my papers. So I don't think the upheavals are really very bad for me.

My darling, I was very, very glad to have your loving letter this morning. It made my work easy for me and it made it far better than it could have otherwise have been. Your love is the most precious thing in the world to me and when I have that, you need not think I need more. I am a very ordinary sort of man my dearest, but with your love I shall also be a happy one and no one can ask more than that. Success, as the world rates it, and outward show are quite agreeable if they come along but they are very much by products which I think come a very long way behind ordinary contentment and happiness. If I can be the same for you then I shall be happy indeed and we shall have all the foundations for a really happy home, and the opportunity of sharing it and spreading it in a modest way to others less fortunate. I know of nothing more satisfactory than that.

And now my dear one I must stop as it is already late. I look forward to seeing you again though it seems a long time ahead. With all my love dear Heart and keep cheerful.

April 24

My darling,

Despite my good resolutions I cannot help just writing you this to say what a heavenly evening it has been. I seem unable to exist without you and I cannot understand how I have survived all these years. Even on a poisonous day like yesterday I knew my work is far better than it has ever been so far. And to-day you simply made the strains roll away. Darling Francesca, how I love you and how I wish I could be with you always.

The group meeting tomorrow night, 'to-night' it will be when you read this, will I am sure make me feel dreadfully ignorant and guilty because I cannot read or write a thing just now although my work with patients is far, far better than it has ever been.

My darling sweetheart I must stop. Once I start on a letter to you I go on thinking of you between every line and word, and I shall end up by being a wreck for want of sleep.

All my love to you Francesca my darling.

Wednesday morning. Good morning my sweetheart. I hope you are well. I am feeling so impatient about seeing you that I have begun to wonder if I was right in thinking so easily that we should let the negotiations for the house take their course, or whether in fact it would not be an advantage for us to have possession of it as soon as possible. If we hurry the contracts it could mean we were free to start working on it—cleaning, repairing, taking in odd bits and pieces. Which is best for you?

April 26

Francesca, my darling,
As I caught a glimpse of you disappearing down the passage before the train doors closed I felt in my heart, There goes my darling; there goes my Life, my All. I love you my dear one.

And that is really all I want to say. Except that I enjoyed this evening so much and feel so refreshed by it that I can hardly reconcile myself to the idea that I really must go to sleep if I am going to do any work at all . . .

April 28

My darling,
I hope, despite the exasperating ending, you enjoyed the party. If I had realized what was happening quicker, I should have stuck to our departure, but T. had offered the lift in front of Mrs Riviere before I could think of an excuse. I couldn't very well say I'd rather miss my train with you than miss it with T.—which I duly did. I hope you got home easily at least. It was only made supportable by the thought that I should be seeing you very soon. I couldn't see how you were getting on but I hope you found it interesting.

As usual I go off into a maze thinking about seeing you tomorrow. You looked lovely to-night; Mrs Riviere said she hoped you were not going to give up music altogether. I think she liked you very much and was genuinely pleased we had come. It was very kind of her to ask us because I rather think it was for our benefit. As she is one of the kingpins of the psycho-analytic world it was a great compliment. Dr Segal is the bright star in the firmament of my generation of psycho-analysts. There is one thing about the psycho-analytic world—we may all be freaks but there are very few I meet who do not seem to me to be intelligent and interesting people; I believe we shall be happy in our social occasions. I have always longed for an intelligent home in which children become accustomed to the company of intelligent people and the sound of good conversation. Perhaps now, through you, I shall have my wish and I hope you will feel, as I think we may, that we can find a social life as well as a happy domestic one.

I thought it a glorious day; from the time we met at Redcourt I enjoyed every second of it and each second was packed with a minute's worth of life. Darling Francesca, I long for our home with a deep yearning. You have made me so happy I hardly know how to live. Dear Darling Francesca, I love you.

April 29

Francesca, my darling love,

I am not really breaking my resolution because I got home very quickly, have had my bath, and just want to write a note to give you tomorrow night.

And what do I want to say so urgently? you will wonder. Well, simply that I love you. My darling I love you. You have done and are still doing something very wonderful to me my dear one. I just feel very happy: so inexpressibly happy. Even my crusted and hardened armour plate of fossilized worry seems to be shaling off each time I see you. I enjoyed every moment of today although I have only the vaguest idea what we did; it is just having you near me.

I feel I can hardly wait for Redcourt. It seems years and years since we thought of finding a house; and yet according to the calendar it cannot be so long.

My dear there is so much I want to say there is no time to say it and I suppose I shall have just have to end up the letter and give it up as a bad job. I am looking forward to tomorrow evening very much indeed although I hardly know how I shall get through the week. I feel as if I were half a person without you. I enjoyed the party with Mrs Riviere very much; I felt she had taken to you and knew at once that I was a very lucky man indeed. I think she has always had something of a liking for me—and she is not exactly easy to please—but yesterday I thought she was convinced that her good opinion of me was proved by your having said 'yes' to me. And I must say I think I am a pretty fine fellow myself, because otherwise I could not have become engaged to you, could I? I really think I must be. In fact there is no doubt about it at all—now.

Francesca my darling sweetheart, goodbye, goodnight my dearest.

May 1

My darling Love,

Just a note to tell you I love you. It seems silly to have to write you a special note to say that but it is so frustrating *not* to say it and anyway why the hell should one be bothered about its being silly or not. So: I love you. I love you.

Sweetheart, don't overdo the work to-night. Someone or other said, when you have too much work to do, don't do it. We both have too much just now. I shall go to bed early tonight and I shall *go to sleep*. Please try to do the same for my sake.

Darling Francesca: unless you have locked your case I shall put this inside it together with a small scattering of kisses.

May 1

Francesca my darling,
It was tantalizing to hear your voice on the phone, tantalizing but sweet all the same. I wish to have you in my arms—but there it is, just a telephone receiver; maddening.

I got back just in time to see Parthenope before she dropped off to sleep—clamouring for more food; she's reached the ravenous stage. She wanted me to tell her "about your boarding school". So I described a school concert while she got through some more food and then she dropped off to sleep. These meetings have a touch of sadness for me as I always feel the barrier of reticence that so often exists. At each week-end she seems more at home and then during the week one is cut off again. I makes me feel that I am not available for the help I would longingly give. She likes to be called my 'big' girl but I always long for her to be my baby still . . .

May 2

Francesca, my sweetheart,
I have been thinking about our marriage. I feel that the beginning of June would be a very good time. I wish it were possible to arrange it in a way that gave us a chance to have a honeymoon, but I think this would be very difficult. From the point of view of work I am inclined to think I ought to work through till about August 8th and make the summer break four weeks—usually it is about five. With a little luck we might then have honeymoon either at Christmas or in Spring. By then we should be a bit settled in and know how things are shaping for us.

I suppose the best day for the marriage and reception would be a Saturday? We shall need to get out invitations pretty soon. I hope above all that in spite of difficulties it will be possible to arrange it so that it will be a really enjoyable thing for others so that they can share a little of the happiness that it means for us. To me it means more than I shall ever be able to say my dearest Francesca.

My dear I find it almost impossible to write to you. I go off into a day-dream at every other line and the result of hours is just this miserable little scrawl of nothing in particular. I am sure I should be thinking of all sorts of business details but somehow they all go clean out of my head. I live a sort of double life; one with my patients trying to keep to the exacting job in hand and also the monthly detail of accounts and such like; and the other centering in the all-absorbing thought of you my dearest. It is no good doing any more except to say that as always I love you my darling Francesca.

With all my love.

May 3

Francesca darling,

If I followed your advice on the phone I should start by writing June 9th followed by a short pause, and then June 9th, with some exclamation marks written in some sort of fiery substance not yet invented alas. Then I think: if this is a dream it is the longest and most marvellous dream I have ever had; if it is not a dream, then I don't know how to contain myself. My goodness, I think, how lovely, how lovely she is. And she has promised to marry *me*. How extraordinary! I must have got myself muddled up with someone else. Whatever shall I do? Will she be very disappointed when she finds out what a dreadfully ordinary person I am? And then I feel rather sad. And then I begin to hope that you like rather ordinary people and that you really know I am ordinary and love me just the same. Is that right? *Do* say it's right. My dearest Francesca, if only I could tell you how I feel. How excited and how nervous. Will you really love me when you know how tired I get when I am fagged out with work? But you must know even now how dull I can be and how tiresome.

I am trying to think of some way we could arrange a honeymoon. I feel it would be a great help if we could manage some time alone together without having to wait too long for it[1] but there is no doubt that the practice is a very serious tie which really dictates our movements very exactingly. But I think it is gradually taking shape—these things have a way of becoming sorted out as one considers the possibilities. It is such a queer business trying to think clearly when for ten hours a day one has the exacting task of being absorbed in the preoccupations of a number of people all of whose holiday arrangements and so on have to depend on those we make ourselves. Not to mention that any of them are liable to commit suicide or some other less spectacular—and in one case *more* spectacular—indiscretion. I have been so much in the air for so long now that I hardly know how the poor things are doing.

Darling, I don't think I've written this any faster. I just have to stop and think how lovely you look. I must be infatuated don't you think? And yet I know I am not. It is just a sober statement of fact; I love seeing your dear face and feel so proud when I feel your arm in mine. Goodnight my darling, darling Francesca. I love you my dearest.

[1] We waited for seven years. In the summer of 1958 we spent a week in Paris.

May 7

Francesca darling,

Just a goodnight note. I am feeling a great mixture of relaxation after the week-end and growing frustration at a return to the week. I do not want to write to you—I want to talk to you and have you in my arms. And I feel a bit grumpy at having to clamber laboriously back to the techniques of living without you . . .

Darling I did enjoy the week-end: even that little taste made me feel as if life has suddenly become more spacious. Dearest as soon as I start writing this I find I get lost in reverie. I don't know how I shall last out the next four weeks. Every now and then I look round and wonder why I can't stay up the whole night packing. Or why some kind person has not already been and offered to buy this house at a sum of money we should approve. But I suppose it will begin to happen. I don't know how we shall spend our last days here. We shall have to live on what we can pack in a few suitcases and have our meals standing up. Dear sweetheart I cannot think how you manage to get any work done at all, leave alone concentrate on it.

Goodbye for the present my darling. I hope you are feeling pretty fit despite your exertions.

With all my love dear Heart.

May 9

Francesca, my darling,

. . . I think I would like to ask Stevie Hall to be best man. Have you any views? He is an old friend, probably the oldest I have.

It was lovely seeing you for our two fleeting meetings. I hardly thought I should see you for the first but since you had not picked up my note I thought I might just meet you coming round from the Clinic. It gave me an excuse for fresh air. And you came like a breath of spring. When I see you I feel, There's my sweetheart. And I am beginning to feel it really must be true. I love you dearest . . .

And now I find I can hardly go on for thinking of you. It seems a terribly long time to have to wait till 5 o'clock tomorrow but I suppose we are luckier than many people in that we see each other as much as we do.

I heard today that someone in the Clinic had said, Just look what a beautiful ring that girl is wearing. It was you. Personally I would say, Just look what a beautiful girl is wearing that ring . . .

May 12

My darling,
I thoroughly enjoyed today's meeting short though it was and even though I manage to get so jittery; I shall improve no doubt. But six years of anxiety centring on the life of a small daughter and how she develops have made me get into a groove of anxiety—trying to be father and mother in one and quite unable to resist the deep urge to do this without feeling worn out . . .

May 17

Francesca my darling,
After our phone call I don't feel that I have anything immediately to write about except to say again that I love you, and to do that with the usual feeling of the inadequacy of words. It needs a full choir, orchestra and organ. However, they are not available at the moment . . .

. . . I so deeply feel that we can build a really happy life and home that it almost makes me afraid. One has seen so many people who seem to have everything with which to build up something really worth while—and then they have just frittered it all away till all that is left is a monument to ineptitude and pettiness. The most ghastly fate, made all the more tragic because it is so unspectacular; just a failure here and another little failure there, multiplied a few hundred times and the trick is done. Well, we must hope to do better; you will have to help me play my part better than I have managed so far . . .

May 18

Francesca my darling,
If I had any strength of will I suppose I should just go to sleep and be content to wake up in the morning but as it is I can only muster enough consideration for you not to ring you up, which I would do if I did not hope you are now in bed, but not enough to refrain from trying to write a few lines to give you in the morning.

I wish everything did not take so long. And sleep takes the most time of all—one must simply sleep so many hours and that is that; there is no way of sleeping in a hurry and getting it done with.

I feel that probably it would be best if you did not have the fatigue of the journey to Iver on Sunday because there is a terrible lot to do and the journey both ways is a lot to pay for what may be a limited amount of benefit. I shall be livid with frustration at not seeing you, and shall work myself into a lather of irritation I do not doubt but I think it will be good for me to make this small sacrifice if it gives you a chance of a little leisure. I do not know how you manage to get through so much and remain so sweet tempered about it. You fill me with admiration and envy till I get quite humiliated at the thought of my selfishness. Tonight passed with maddening speed and I felt I had wasted the fleeting moments not only for myself but also for you. And now as I try to write this I gaze at your photo and wish it was you. I am sorry my dear; but I wish I could make *you* feel how much *I* feel what you do for me.

Well, my dear, it won't be long after I have handed you this that I shall be able to see you again and if I can't do much else I shall at least be able to look at you and indeed that is a great deal.

Francesca darling, Darling, my dear love, goodbye for the present . . . Saturday morning in the train. I feel as excited as I always feel at the thought I shall see you soon. This train shakes so much I cannot write . . .

Good-morning my dearest.

May 19

Francesca my darling,

. . . Ought we sometime to think of what guests at the Reception might want to mix with others there unknown to them? Or do we just let them mill around and think what odd people the others are and how odd we must be to know such queer fish? I think I ought to keep a list of guests to get the names well into my mind beforehand. It is good to study these details because so often the difference between an indifferent show and a good show depends on some such little preparation, even though on the actual occasion it may not seem to count for much

The thought inspires me to embark on another instalment of Bion history. So here goes: I hope you don't mind?

Roy Bion, 'Noah', belongs to the Rupert Bion outfit. My Uncle Rupert was married to my Aunt Alice. He became enormously wealthy, by Bion standards, but lost it all in the end. He was an indigo planter in India and could have ended very wealthy but was so annoyed with Congress and Ghandi that he preferred to go down fighting rather than sell out at a profit which he might have done. He was a very stout genuine soul with all the Anglo-Indian merchant's ignorance of culture and indifference to everything except hard work and personal comfort. His sons were Euston—I think they must have meant Eustace but got mixed up with the railway station—Ken, Roy and Laurie. His daughter was a minx of the name of Gladys. I only knew them when in England since I never went back to India after eight.

Whenever I came across them I was impressed by the atmosphere of luxury and indescribable chaos. Euston and Ken, as befits young men at Trinity, Cambridge, and New College, Oxford, were painfully ashamed of their family and painstakingly determined to lick it into shape. Uncle Rupert was humorously charmed by an appreciative awareness of the fact that he himself was the source of their greatest embarrassment. He recognized that he was the formidable barrier to any real advance in the social scale. When I was about ten I spent a few days at their house in Bedford. At the time Ken and Euston were pursuing two young women of the Bedford aristocracy and were doing their best to hide from these young women the dreadful nature of the home to which they had perforce to invite these elegant nymphs. As I remember them they must have been two quite ordinary, quite nice, well dressed girls but beyond that I can say nothing as even then it was fascinating to me to observe the contortions, the painful angular manoeuvres to which Euston and Ken were reduced at lunch and subsequently when they were present with the two ladies. My uncle in turn must have observed *me* for he tackled me, when he found himself alone with me, something after this style as one man of the world to another.

"Well, Wilfred, and how do you like my house?" Here he paused and as he puffed wheezily in his chair looked at me through his screwed up little eyes with a quizzical expression.

"I think it very nice, Uncle", I replied, secretly awe-struck at the luxury.

"Mm— Euston tells me that it is not in very good taste. Of course I don't understand these things, but what do you think Wilfred?"

"I don't know, Uncle. I think it's awfully, well awfully nice, Uncle."

"Mm—but you know Wilfred, Euston says that at Trinity they would not think much of it. Trinity is a very fine place, you know Wilfred. They wouldn't have anyone like you or me there; at least they might have you but I don't think they'd like me there."

This would be beyond me so I swung my legs and said nothing. He went on, "Euston says we ought to have another car. He says that a Rolls Royce and a Sunbeam aren't enough but I tell him he has his own car. Now what do you think Wilfred? I've always heard the Rolls Royce was a good car".

"What would you do with another, Uncle?"

"That's just what I say to Euston, Wilfred", my uncle beamed back at me.

"Perhaps, Uncle, you could tow it behind the Rolls—like a sort of dinghy, Uncle"', I replied entering into the spirit of the thing.

"'He says I ought to get up earlier in the morning. What do you think?"

"I like lying in bed, Uncle."

"I can see, Wilfred, that you and I would get on famously together. What is the use, I always say, of getting up when you are on holiday and there is no work to do?"

And so on.

Euston was a nice lad but I think he had the most resounding inferiority I have ever come across. The result was that when war came he had to go into nothing less than the Horse Guards. For a couple of years the Horse Guards never went into action though they were in France—it was no war for gee-gees.

His desire to fight got the better of his inferiority, so, fed up with burying the dead, he joined what was then the Royal Flying Corps and was finally killed in action.

Ken who was a very handsome man was, I always thought, rather an unpleasant one, selfish and vain and rather unkind. He was killed in action in the Sherwood Foresters after winning the Military Cross.

Noah came next. A dreamy, rubber-faced lad with an expression like a cocker spaniel pup. He salvaged the wreckage of the indigo plantations, worked till he felt he had made ample money to make further work unnecessary and packed up. He never had any use for work anyway. The comfortable and unintelligent life for him every time. He married someone who makes him shave and dress but does not otherwise bother him I imagine. I forget her name; it may be Maud.

Laurie married a Jewess called Yvonne. She struck me as a tiresomely alert and unattractive woman. I don't know what has happened to him. They divorced, which was in no way surprising. It must have been wretched to be married to either of them.

Gladys was a nasty little minx who looked and behaved like a gipsy. At one time she went on the films and appeared in a crowd scene in *The Wreck of the Titanic*. It has always been one of my most pleasant thoughts imagining Gladys sitting amidst the ruins of a cardboard Titanic soulfully singing, 'Nearer my God to Thee'. She must be knocking around somewhere but I won't have anything to do with her. The last I heard of her was when she left her father to it when he was dying in Weston-Super-Mare. I went down to see the old man just after she had left. He was in bed and his heart was conking out. He told me the doctor had seen him and said he should go to a nursing home but he wouldn't unless the doctor could promise that he would be dead within the week. He couldn't. He left, telling him that on no account was he to leave his room. No sooner had he gone than my uncle, who was not impressed by life since his wife had died some few years before when they were in Australia—a long and painful illness of some kind—skipped out of bed and got into a cab. In this he went to the local undertaker and arranged for his funeral. "I couldn't", he said, "get Gladys to do this as it would have upset her."

When I left him I thought I had better go and find out if all really was settled before I returned to Town. The undertaker I duly found, a very much shaken man, who indeed confirmed that everything was fixed up. He wound up by saying in an awe-struck voice that my uncle had haggled over the cost of the funeral and had finally beaten him down to do the whole bag of tricks for £20. Poor man; it must have been an unnerving experience trying to maintain his professional unctuosity while arguing finance with the prospective corpse. I went back to my uncle's hotel to say goodbye as I had to be back in hospital. He kept his sense of humour to the end and was, I think, amused at my somewhat nonplussed embarrassment at a final farewell. I couldn't very well wish him a pleasant trip and yet that was about all his manner allowed to be appropriate.

Now my darling, I must stop this drivel. It helps to pass the time till June 9th. I love you always my darling.

My dear love, goodbye for the present.

May 23

Francesca my dearest,

Even the telephone has a most disturbing effect on me sometimes, particularly when you are using the other end of it. I am now confronted by a white piece of paper instead of a black plastic phone receiver and don't find the change makes me feel any cooler or calmer.

Darling Francesca, words are very unsatisfactory things sometimes and this is one of them. If I could hear you speaking them it would be a different matter—provided it was from somewhere nearer to me.

I suppose I ought to pull myself together and write business; I shall try. The reception: Jack Drummond[1] is a very nice man. He is of course a very good biochemist but he has also travelled all over the world as far as I can make out and done it in all sorts of conditions . . .

May 26

Francesca my darling,
In the train coming back Parthenope wanted to smell my tobacco. She said she did not like it. I said, in tones of surprise, *Don't* you? She said, No; but then of course I am a woman! As she was utterly serious she could not understand the sensation this caused among the other passengers.

. . . I fixed up with Brown's Hotel as I told you. I think it was the best arrangement and though expensive I felt we had avoided extravagance on the one hand and on the other the sort of parsimony that can make people feel that an occasion that should be happy and is important, has been turned into a rather uneasy congregation of people wondering if they ought not to club together to provide money for a couple who have hit on this method of raising the wind. I don't think any but the most uncharitable would think either extreme had been achieved: and let us hope none of them would be present . . .

June 5

My darling love,
Just a very short note to say how much I love you and how much I appreciate the enormous amount of work you are doing. I feel terribly in a backwater pegging along with patients exactly as if nothing was happening . . .

The new owner of the house was round this evening. He seemed a very decent sort of man and quite pleased with his purchase. I think he has reason to be and it may suit him. For myself I am more than ever relieved at being rid of what I am convinced is going to be a liability before many years are out.

Darling sweetheart I love you and hope I shall make you very happy.

June 9

Francesca, darling love,
My last letter to you before our marriage must be simply to say I love you my darling and—you make me feel so proud.

[1] See p. 46.

It is hard to realize how much this means. June 9th 1951. For ever and ever my dear darling I love you. I hope that you will be happy whatever may come our way, and that I may make you so.

Redcourt

To Bournemouth July 9

My darling,

. . . I wanted badly to do some serious psycho-analytic work but I found myself unbelievably shy of starting it. I really have become terribly out of the way of reading it, not that I ever did much in that way at any time. There are few psycho-analytic writers who write clearly and those, except Freud, are not always the best psycho-analysts. Still, one ought I think constantly to revise and keep what has been written, by a few of the best at least, well in mind. How this is to be done, with the general reading that I also consider essential, no one knows.

. . . The house is very empty without you and Parthenope—not that she makes her presence felt at this hour—and I shall go to bed early.

Sunday afternoon. I have written my short piece about Rickman[1] and that must go off tomorrow . . . I would have written something not banal but there is a convention in these things which must be adhered to—at least it is risky to depart from it very much.

Well, my dear wife, this house is lonely without you. I would look up as I write this and see you opposite but alas it is not to be, and a fortnight is a very long time to wait. It is nice writing, my dear wife: Francesca my darling wife: how I long to—but it does not bear thinking about.

I hope you are having a fine day. It is lovely here . . . there is a good breeze, warm and caressing. And there has been plenty of sun. If it has been like that at Bournemouth then I hope you have had a good day on the beach and feel the cobwebs all blown away. Get well pickled in the sea too. I think it makes one's skin really fit to have the stimulation of the salt water and sea air. I have no doubt Parthenope is revelling in it . . .

[1] John Rickman died on July 1.

July 9

My darling wife,
My darling Mrs Bion: How are you now my dearest Mrs Bion? It makes me angry and sad to think that owing to my stupidity over stamps you will not have had my Sat-Sun letter this morning. But I hope there will not be any more delays.

I very unfairly had two letters from you this morning and was so glad to get them that I couldn't bear to open them as I wanted somewhere absolutely private where I could read them without any rush. Thank you for them my darling wife. They were very welcome and interesting. It makes me hope that you are having an enjoyable and happy time.

It also makes me feel more than ever that I would come down to Bournemouth for the next week-end but even if you were able to arrange for me at the hotel, which I suppose is unlikely, I feel troubled about expense. I suppose it is irrational to be disturbed over the way they go on delaying settlement of the Homestead but it does bother me.

. . . I am very interested in your news of our daughter—shivering with cold and sniffling has never been accepted by her as anything against swimming.

Darling Mrs Bion; yes, I think it looks very nice. So does she. Sleep well dearest—if this reaches you at night.

Your loving husband.

July 9

My darling Wife,
The sound of your dear voice has really put some life into me in a most magical way . . . It has even had the effect of making me get out my own group paper[1] and look at it. There really is a big difficulty about this. I think that to psycho-analyse patients properly—and I think I am doing this quite well at the moment—one has to keep one's touch concentrated on that sort of outlook; one should not do something too close to it—either analysis only or else something quite different, a complete change. They say you should never play a game with a stationary ball, like golf, when you are trying to play well in a game with a moving ball, like tennis. It is something of that sort. Anyhow I often feel after throwing myself into group work that I do very bad analysis just after it. Of course it may be illusory.

The other paper I spoke about was an expansion of my member-

[1] 'Group Dynamics: a Re-View'. The International Journal of Psycho-Analysis, Vol. XXXIII, Part II, 1952. Also, *New Directions in Psycho-Analysis*, Tavistock Publications Ltd., 1955.

ship paper.[1] This is I believe a *really* good paper and it very badly needs expansion and publication. Probably I had better concentrate on that at least till the summer holiday. However there is no harm in keeping the thread of the other in mind so I can get off to a flying start. It is maddening when one's interest shifts from a subject too much.

My darling I love you: I can't tell you how much better I feel for hearing the sound of your voice on the phone. I feel jealous and envious of Bournemouth to think you are there and I'm so far away . . .

P.S. Since June 9th 1951, your husband. How satisfying it is to write that. Your husband. My darling wife Francesca.

July 10

My darling wife,
This must be a very short note as it is late and tomorrow is an early morning and late night. The only merit of it is that I hope it will make the time go faster. At least it is Tuesday night—but really! only two days gone!

I am just back from supper with Ken Rice. We met at Maison de France. Quite a good meal for a change but how I grudged the time. I was sorry because I like him, but at the moment it reminds me only too poignantly of batchelor days so I felt ungrateful.

I have been trying to sort out income tax in intervals between patients to-day. Really one wonders if ever one will have time to do any real work. And yet when one is hopelessly in arrears with routine Income Tax stuff and already feels desperately tired, it is hard to know what to do. I feel guilty but I am already doing a 50-hour week of patients and that is nearly too much in itself.

I have come reluctantly to the conclusion that I shall absolutely have to put up my fees after this summer. I am sure I am charging far too litle. It is a very great nuisance but it is doing neither me nor my patients much good. People not one half as good as I am are charging more . . .

July 11

My darling wife,
Just as I thought the postman would not be in time he came, so off I went to Town with your letter snug in my pocket.

[1] 'The Imaginary Twin'.

When I read your account of the early morning I reminded myself that holidays are only work disguised so as to look different from work!

Needless to say your suggestion of the week-end agitates me. I would love to come especially if I could get off on Friday night. It would help to cut short this intolerable pause I suppose; I never knew time drag so horribly. It would be awful if it made the remaining time seem to go even more slowly—if such a thing is possible.

I have been to a business meeting of the Institute. The first ¾ hour was spent in talks by various people in memory of Rickman. Rather stiff and too formal for the most part but Money-Kyrle spoke well—he who wrote the obituary in *The Times*.

Darling wife, I love you dearest. I don't want to go on writing so-called news. I quite enjoyed the meeting but I spent most of it thinking complacently and very happily about you. Two people told me how well I looked and I knew they both knew it was you. This gave me much pleasure. But—my goodness how the days drag. It is too painful to realize this is only Wednesday. I really thought the fortnight would be soon over, or told myself so till I believed it. I know better now and cannot keep up the pretence . . .

July 12

My darling love,
You cannot think what a thrill it is for me at the beginning of the day to see your handwriting on the envelope in the box—and with what depression and anxiety I approach it in case it is not there. I say to myself, Of course there won't be one today because the posts will be irregular. Or, she may not have time. Or, well, why *should* she write every day anyway? And then . . . ah! there it is; I can see something in the box even through the glass doors. I am writing this immediately when I have just opened your letter, in the short space between two patients, but have only read the first sentence . . .

I am sorry the weather has been poor as I believe it would be very good for you to get plenty of sun and air—also sea bathes. Also I agree with you that an absence of me is doing you no good. *I* am the medicine you need all right. Plenty of me, day and night, for ever. We shall have to arrange it . . .

Well I have just spoken to you on the phone and that has put everything out of my head except the thought of our meeting. Truly I never felt a fortnight could possibly be such a weary agony of waiting. I don't know how I shall last out the next week. This one seems to have been almost as much as I could stand and heaven knows it has been easy enough . . .

July 18

Francesca my darling,
It is *still* Wednesday: I never knew it go on being Wednesday for so long before. And I sit about filled with the most gloomy forebodings feeling that the house never will be sold or, worse still, that the bank, the solicitors and the agents between them will get all the money. I don't quite know what lesson one should learn from all this but I am sure there is something. The assistant bank manager said to me, "These solicitors are *all* rogues, *all* of them. You may have paid for the house but who knows if the vendor has the money yet." I thought he might have added banks to solicitors but did not say so.

I think as you do about children. Anyhow I feel that we could at least do our best to make a happy home which people who do not love each other cannot do. Whether our best would be good enough no one can tell but the idea of it is thrilling . . . It is tragic how often parents hinder rather than help the development of their children: and the child is always so helpless, so little able to contribute to a harmonious home. Like as not it quite unconsciously sets about making mischief or difficulty.

I have been doing some of my group paper in the interval when a patient was away. It is not good as it stands but it may be possible to expand it into something worthwhile. It has possibilities. As usual I find myself brought up short by the lack of time to do all one would like. And yet if I had more time I should probably do what everyone with time seems to do—waste it. I think really I get through a great deal of work but I am apt to forget that I have done ten hours of patients and wonder why my mind is not fresh. Luckily I have a great capacity for being lazy and I think this saves me from overwork. Rickman I don't think ever attached enough importance to this, perhaps by temperament, and I think he wasted himself very badly. He had a very good brain but I think for the last ten years there was a falling off. He did not himself realize it luckily. The surprising thing is that so few others noted it either though it was very marked . . .

. . . I find I cannot contain my impatience. Two more days might be two months I feel it such a drag. It is as if it were such a frustration that I can hardly look forward to Saturday. I love you my darling wife . . .

July 19

Francesca darling,
I was very glad to hear your voice to-night as I haven't had a letter but it was all too short a talk. Also I was so pleased at hearing you that I could not think what depression you were referring to—it had all gone at the sound of your voice.

. . . My dear, the nearer it comes to Saturday the more I feel I can't bear the long wait. Really I do not know quite what you have done to me: I seem totally incapable of getting on without you! And I am sure you will think the house is a pig sty and quite topsy-turvy.

It has not felt a satisfactory day's work today. I think patients are all very much in need of a holiday as I am and it is difficult to keep a track of them all. They all seem to want to stop treatment, even the most unsuitable for ending. Since one feels like stopping oneself, it is not very easy to deal with.

July 20

Francesca my darling,
Just a note which I hope will be in time to reach you before you leave Bournemouth. It is to send you my love and to wish you a very pleasant and comfortable journey and to remind you that even if you don't you will soon be having the outstanding pleasure of seeing ME! Even so you will not I fear have such an exciting and altogether stupendous pleasure as I shall be having because I shall be meeting YOU. Now isn't that nice for me?

Darling, darling Francesca. How I long to meet 'my women' (as Dr Heimann called you, rather amusingly I thought). Give our daughter a kiss from me.

My sweetheart: what ages you have been away. Tell the driver of the train to get a move on please. I shall be seeing you soon, you know.

July 21

Francesca my darling,
You wouldn't think it but I have already been writing this letter for half an hour. And yesterday evening I couldn't even get this far.

Very shortly I shall be setting out to meet my darling wife . . . I keep thinking I am at Waterloo trying to pierce through the crowd of passengers coming. My goodness where are you? I hope you haven't missed the train. Surely by this time I should have caught a glimpse of you? If you had caught the train—Really it is terribly careless of you; I believe you *have* missed the train damn it! You might have known I wouldn't be able to bear it if you—Ah!—she hasn't missed it! Bless her! my darling girl. My darling, darling girl. What a time it takes to get through this crowd. And even when I do I won't really be able to kiss her.

Darling this is hopeless. I can't stand it and I'm off to Waterloo. I ought to have got the Hoover out or gone and picked some raspberries or something. It's like waiting for school term to end. Or leave to come due at the front when a battle is on and you think you may get killed or, worse still, trip up and sprain your ankle and miss your turn that way. It's like, well, I suppose it's only like one thing on earth—meeting Francesca when she is your darling, darling wife.

There is *nothing* else like it. Only that . . .

1952

Redcourt

To the Mayday Hospital August 13

My darling wife,

. . . I feel more and more how happy and fortunate I am, even if it does mean the most agonizing frustration too.

I had a pleasant surprise and relief to-day as my patient—'the' one—turned up and was not quite so virulent as before; but what was better, when his father arrived, he started off by saying that both he and his wife were *amazed* at the change in the boy. He said he was kind, considerate and with a marked sense of responsibility, and that they had never known him like that before. I told him I was very glad to hear it because of course what I saw was all the anxiety and conflict and hate, and that although I could *deduce* progress that was not the same as an independent witness. Now aren't you pleased? I am. It is one of the things that goes towards making one feel that all the sweat and blood of this business is well worth it—not that one always has such appreciative parents. It is a great load off my mind and it is very gratifying to me because it makes me feel, *What a clever* husband you've got! . . .

The patient's father, by the way, had seen *The Times* announcement and gave his congratulations.[1]

Darling I can't bear going on writing this as all the things I want to say won't come out in a staid and respectable manner as befits a husband married to such a clever and beautiful wife . . .

August 14

Francesca my darling,

. . . I had the best session yet with my problem child and although there were extraneous reasons for it, it is also a sign of good work here. My darling sweetheart this is all you. If it were not for the thought of your love for me I don't believe I could cure anybody or anything—certainly not in the state of mind I've been in for the last month. I've been terribly anxious and worried and I have yearned for you day and night till I felt I could hardly bear it, but I think all the same I have been able to do, and even do well, the things I have had to do. And I feel extremely happy. My darling I hope you will

[1] Julian was born on July 30.

feel blessed in your family. I hope you will feel it is as a source of deep joy and happiness that nothing can take away from you no matter what anxieties and troubles may be in store—we couldn't do without them either I am sure . . . If only I could have known you earlier! And now there's Julian, bless him! Well, I shall have to get to know him—and you, because I think you have changed you know. Anyway I shall have to look into the matter . . .

1953

Redcourt

To Angmering August 4

My darling,

. . . My worry is whether the house will turn it all into a busman's holiday.[1] It would be a great help to the children if they have a chance of having you to themselves. I curse myself for this arrangement of holiday because I feel both I and my patients are going through with it but without any real drive—as if feeling it a waste of time. And a number have gone anyhow so it would have been better to quit. I shall try to use the gaps in my practice for reading or writing but to-day at least I felt I lacked resilience or interest.

. . . Well my love I think of you all the time. Please give my love and kisses and a hug to Parthenope and a, well whatever he calls it, to Julian. It seems queer to have a son and daughter. I really feel quite a family man now.

Goodnight my love: I love you. But how I hate writing letters . . .

[1] We rented a house for a month by the sea.

1955

Redcourt

To the Mayday Hospital June 12

My darling,
Just a line to let you know all goes well here. Parthenope has been playing with Julian the whole time so he has been quiet enough—if quiet is the right word. Your mother gave him an excellent answer when he asked when you would be back: she said you had got to wait till the baby was big enough. It had the blessed merit of being true, comprehensible to him, and satisfying as well . . .

You are always in my thoughts my brave sweetheart.

June 17

My darling,
. . . I have been thinking the matter over and have come to the conclusion that Nicola is the most beautiful baby in the world[1]. It's this hospital business that gets me down: I've just remembered it was the same with Julian—an agonizing and indefinable postponement.

He said to me he wanted his Mummy and then—*don't* go to work Daddy. So he wants us both which is very satisfactory . . .

Geneva[2]

July 24

My darling,
I had a very good and easy journey and now of course I am more than ever sorry you are not here—Nicola and all. The children would love it, and if Julian had been able to keep his eyes open he would have been thrilled to bits by the airport at London. It is a vast place and the bus ran in by a long underground tunnel that reminded me of the Mersey tunnel. The lighting in the reception halls was wonderfully effective and I think owes something to the Festival of Britain

[1] She was born on June 13.
[2] He was attending an International Psycho-Analytical Congress.

artists. The plane was a turbo-jet and the take-off and the whole flight was extremely smooth even if it did not live up to being 'without vibration' quite as they advertised. But it was so steady that it gave me a feeling of confidence that I have not had before in flying. We rose very fast to 17,000 feet and 300 miles an hour. In 20 minutes we were over Brighton and in another 20 minutes over France; Paris—Dijon—a snooze, and we were circling Geneva airport. I felt a bit tatty by the time I was thrown out of the bus, but all went smoothly and I soon became aware that my misgivings arose from my expecting English service. By four o'clock I had my luggage and was clear. Of course I wondered how on earth I was to get to the hotel and if there would be a room. And of course nothing could be simpler. A row of taxis—unlike Croydon—a swift ride for 1fr.50 (about 3/-) and there I was wondering if the hotel was open at such an hour. A room? Certainly m'sieur: number 309 . . .

. . . at 8.15 I rang down for my 'café complet' which is included. I had hardly settled back on my pillows before the waiter was there. Two fresh rolls and a croissant, very good butter, apricot jam and lots of coffee and milk. And all most fresh and appetising. There is a writing desk and, as you can see, notepaper etc. It seemed to me my only chance of writing was to do it now while Melanie presumably thinks I am asleep—once I showed myself, I felt sure, she would not let me off re-writing my paper. Even now I suspect she will send someone to rout me out on the grounds I have had quite enough sleep to go on with . . .

I must say I feel deeply sorry you aren't here. Honestly I believe it would be a holiday and a rest to you if you simply stayed here and looked after Nicola while I coped with Julian and Parthenope. The cleanliness, the service and efficiency alone raise one's morale. I believe we should aim at something like this next year willy-nilly[1]. I am *sure* we could find something which would be as easy, no, far easier a holiday than Farringford[2] and an infinitely simpler and more comfortable journey. Although I haven't poked my nose out of doors yet this has brought home to me in full force that England is no place for a holiday—unless you stay at home and that is no holiday for you. How I long for you to be here . . .

I must find a way of explaining to M.K. that I need sleep and then use it for writing! Psycho-analysis all day and psycho-politics all night, preferably in a room with all the windows shut, cigarettes alight, and a fire, is more than my constitution was built for. I shall

[1] We went to Lake Garda.
[2] Once Tennyson's house, at Freshwater on the Isle of Wight.

add to the fug with a cigar and if that does not clear the room I shall say I must go to write my October paper[1]; there is some truth in this anyway. And now my dear I must deal with Herr-monsieur, cher docteur-med or whatever his title should be. I feel a brute but I am sure he will be relieved too. With all my love my darling. I think of you always. And it is nearly half Sunday gone. With many many kisses.

July 24

Francesca darling,

. . . As soon as I went down to post the letter to you, there at the barrier was Elliott Jaques, and there by his side Melanie. So we had lunch. And very good too: an artichoke, a mixed grill consisting of sweetbreads, veal, chop, pork sausage, fennel, kidney and tournedos excellently cooked. Then raspberries and a coffee ice cream. And the sun blazed and a cool breeze blew and the Rhône dashed along in front of us.

We then had a drive for some miles along Lake Geneva, beautiful in the sun with all the families out in their chic. The most amazing sight is a fountain which throws the water 270 feet into the sky—a remarkable feat of hydraulic engineering. And so back to an afternoon rest . . .

Then the reception. In a very big hall in the best hotel. There must have been about a thousand people. Masses of all sorts and my reeling brain saw Argentinians and Brazilians and one Mexican and—some talking broken English and some broken French but all, I gather, had been greatly stimulated by my articles, my 'sporadic' articles one of them said. I felt like a stuffed cod served with hot butter sauce and looked it. I *had* to drink, and the more I drank the more of course I sweated. Many friends say what a pity you aren't here. Of course. And so do I, many times.

M.K. and Elliott interest me. There is no doubt of the close collaboration: and why not? It does not do to think you can be a failure in this world and get away with it. At last we left. The reflections in the water, the floodlit fountain and the rushing Rhône looked very fine. Shops are likewise but *very, very* expensive.

I think of you always and there is much I would like to talk to you about on the spot while fresh in the mind . . .

[1] 'Development of Schizophrenic Thought'.

July 25

My darling,

I have a moment so had better seize it. M.K. and Elliott are at the Congress but I have stayed on the pretext that I want to review my paper; so I do, but I want to stay away from the Congress more. The morning's session was not as bad as it might have been but whether that was because I wore my linen trousers and terylene shirt, and was more comfortable in consequence, or whether on account of the excellence of the papers I would not like to determine; more I suspect the former than the latter. I hate listening to lectures anyway. There was one fool of a woman who talked on, but knew nothing about, schizophrenia. She was allowed 30 minutes; she read a paper of 60 minutes gabbled so as to fit it into 45. And Melanie said her piece and was pleased with its reception. Augusta Bonnard (Mrs Brunner) thinks, says M.K., that I am charming. Obviously the old spells still work you see. I strolled back past shops and am convinced there is nothing I can buy here which would not be both uninteresting and expensive. The only local objects would be a watch for Parthenope and a cuckoo clock for Julian. Or, just a cuckoo clock for *us* which would amuse the children . . .

I decided to economize by having a glass of beer and a sandwich for lunch: bill 9frs.90, which according to my reckoning is close on £1.

Later. Well, anyhow now it is Monday night. I am just back after a trip out with Elliott and Melanie in his car, to a lake-side restaurant for supper. During the afternoon there was a thunderstorm in the neighbourhood, with a few drops of rain here, so by the time Elliott rang me up, at about 6.15 p.m., it had become nice and cool. The drive, of a few kilometres, was nothing in particular—a wide 4-lane speed road with glimpses of the lake—and the restaurant unpretentious. It was quite a nice little meal; trout meunière, escallope of veal, an ice sweet and coffee; a local white wine, uninteresting but not vinegar. It cost about 25/- each which I think a good Soho standard; better than my beer and sandwich at least. The conversation I now feel was a bore, but am a bit guilty at thinking so. Melanie is extremely demanding. I suppose it is because she has had so many attacks and so little genuine happiness in her life but I always feel sucked dry; I don't know quite how it is. I think she fishes for a compliment, gets it, rejects it and then says, "But all the same I think he" (or she or it or them) "is really quite friendly to me". I am supposed to be in a state of nerves about my paper. In fact I don't give a damn about it. But she likes to reassure me. Later she will want to stop me from being conceited about it.

But enough of this. I am hoping to have a letter from you tomorrow. Indeed I kept looking for one today although I knew there couldn't have been one. I feel I have been away for at least ten days although this time two days ago I had only just left you . . .

After a little more acquaintance with Geneva I am not so sorry you are not here—it is so obvious that if one comes abroad at all Geneva is *not* the place, and except for income tax rebate it is a waste of time to mix it up with a congress. Congresses for London—abroad for holidays.

I suppose I had better stop if I'm going to be in a fit state to do my 20 minutes tomorrow. Melanie asked after Nicola and spoke very warmly of you saying how well you got on with everyone and how much everyone liked you. It always gives me great happiness when I hear my wife loved and admired—and it makes me feel very warm to Melanie, even if, for some reason, I'm a bit cross at the time. I have to be at the Congress all day tomorrow and a Cantonal Reception in the evening, sweating and hot in my suit, so I don't expect I shall be able to write at any length. But I shall try to write something and at least to say how the paper went off and how much I love you . . .

July 26

My darling,

I'm starting this before breakfast partly as I may not have time later and partly to let Elliott and Melanie get off to the Congress without me. I feel a bit battered at the moment. To be a bit irreverent, it all reminds me of stories a friend of mine told me about Marlene Dietrich who, said he, was surrounded by a squad of the most beautiful—teutonically beautiful that is—young men, who leapt—that was the only movement permitted I gather—to fulfil her slightest wish, and to beat off any would-be intruder. If Melanie had her way, and she has a lot of it, she would make the whole Klein group quite ridiculous in everyone's eyes. I have an excuse in my 'nervousness' so mean to arrive by myself on foot. I may be wrong, of course. But I don't think so.

I hope to find a letter from you this morning when I go down shortly. There was another thunderstorm last night and I see the streets are still wet. As it's a totally indoors occupation here I welcome it as a way of keeping cool. I hope the poor things who are having holidays in the mountains like it.

Evening. I have half an hour before a ghastly evening of reception and Argentinian party. There is still no letter so I shall not hear till tomorrow now. I hope you and the children have had better luck with my efforts.

The afternoon was a success but I feel a bit flat partly because it was pretty evident that no one understood a word I was talking about. M.K. says they will do later: perhaps. First B., who is a rogue, spoke for 29 minutes instead of 20 allotted; then Segal for 27 minutes instead of 20 allotted; then I, who spoke for 19—a bit fast. In the discussion B. attacked me quite rightly for the clinical material, but it gave me the chance to explain what my paper was about and to explain a part of a part of an interpretation, and I gather from one or two people that it made an enormous difference to those who previously had been puzzled.

I feel most reluctant to go to this infernal cantonal reception . . . I don't want to grumble because in fact I would feel churlish and stupid if I didn't go, and I should also feel I was missing something.

I must go my darling. I think of you and the children all the time. I hope all is well with you. Please kiss them for me . . .

Later. Well I'm back and as it is only 11.30 I shall jot down the evening's news. The rooms for the reception were in beautiful gardens with as beautiful a view of the lake. Snacks and drinks all very pleasant. When it was over we found we could stay there and have a meal and this M.K., Elliott and I did. And an excellent meal it was. I had a very well cooked sole with mushrooms, a tournedos and vegetables, and a coupe Jaques in honour of Jaques and my Tummy. White + red wine all excellent and one franc *less* than the previous evening, which is surprising. Then we went to the Argentine party. It was held in the flat of an Argentine couple. Coffee: more drink: a trolley load of fruit salads most exotically decorated, and in the background through the windows a view of the lake aflame with lights of Geneva across on the other side. Some dancing went on to Argentinian music. Then a psycho-analyst, a Spaniard, sang a series of flamenco songs. The scene was attractive and went well with the belly-aching wail and the thrum of the guitar—the lake and its lights through the windows and the very Mexican-Exhibition-looking women about the floor and looped around window seats. Melanie said, What a pity Francesca is not here. Which I echoed with all my heart. At last home, and very glad to be back. I will not pretend I am not very disappointed to have had no word whatever of you or the children since I left on Saturday night. I love you and them too dearly not to be upset, but perhaps it is only Croydon post office . . .

July 27

My darling,

I went off duly to listen to Gillespie at 9.0 a.m. and then stayed on for some discussion. I had a shock when calling for letters to find a telegram which I tore open and was relieved to find it was only from an ex-patient. I feel very sleepy as I didn't sleep much at night and this is a sleepy town. Segal, who was apparently at school here, says it is a wretched place, always steamy, hot and cloudy. At the moment it is fine, but otherwise it lives up to her description.

Some man wanted me to join them in a group therapy session at lunch to-day. I want to cut it: it is just the day for a quiet lunch entirely by myself I feel.

Later. However, I went: and I felt that I was a silly ass because it turned out to be a very crowded and uncomfortable indoor lunch with people who didn't know much about it. I was however listened to with flattering attention and I had a very good omelette and a beer, and that is something. But at the moment, which is midnight, the main thing is that I have had a letter from you. When I came back after the last paper of the Congress there it was. I gather you sent it on Monday so it seems extraordinary that I have had to wait till Wednesday evening before getting it. But it has made me feel quite different. I have really felt very worried and that damned telegram made me have a nasty shock. It is a great relief that all was going on ordinarily and I am ashamed to say I even felt a little bit glad you missed me.

To go back to the story: I went to the papers chiefly to hear Money-Kyrle and Rosenfeld. Money-Kyrle was very gentlemanly and Elliott thought it was good for them all to see how an Old Etonian died in the last ditch so to speak. Rosenfeld's was the last in the Congress and I thought it good.

I joined Elliott and M.K. and he drove us to the Beau-Rivage where we had a beer on a terrace lined with tiny pink lorraine begonias. Then ten minutes to tidy up at the hotel where I found your letter thank God. I had walked back at midday before the group therapy lunch but had only found notice of the telegram. I hadn't even heart to buy some magnificent cherries[1] in the market place on the island in the Rhône.

Then Elliott drove M.K. and me to a château on the outskirts of Lausanne—about an hour's drive. This trip was to a dinner given to the Congress by Raymond de Saussure—some 800-900 guests. I was

[1] His favourite fruit.

curious to see what it was all about as it seemed a somewhat generous venture and M.K. had said that I must go because if de Saussure did it, it was bound to be good. Well, after a somewhat tantalizing drive on which one only had occasional glimpses, from an arterial road, of the lake, the moon, and Mont Blanc, we reached the village which was dominated by this castle. The castle turns out to be de Saussure's brother's and has been in the family since about 1600 or earlier. We had police to control the traffic and all the parking was done with no fuss or trouble. Then we walked about 100 yards up to the main gate of the castle through which we entered a truly magnificent courtyard which was dominated by the keep and high tower—an affair of massive proportions and very awe-inspiring. We climbed the stairs and entered a big hall with ceiling painted with coats of arms. From this we walked through an ante-room to a terrace along which was set out long dining tables in the open air with the lake spread below us in the evening glow beneath the moon. The terrace went down in stages for some 60 yards or more and tables were set for the guests beneath trees festooned with small electric light bulbs. Elliott, M.K. and I sat ourselves down at the tables on the highest level outside the ante-room—the serfs, I told Melanie to her pleasure, would be at the lower tables. The meal was simple—a small cheese soufflé, a cold pie with engaging but not particularly memorable etceteras, and an iced sweet and coffee. There was plentiful agreeable white and red wine and the only marring feature was that Melanie fell from her seat and hurt herself. She was not as much shaken as I feared and I hope not much hurt. She seemed to recover very well.

No speeches but de Saussure walked round amongst the guests and was very deservedly clapped, with some health-drinking of course. By this time there were sounds of music and we broke up and moved indoors.

The main hall was cheerful with people, informally but nicely dressed, and I soon discovered that the music came from two Swiss in very gay scarlet costumes, playing traditional Swiss airs on small but very powerful concertinas. One was on the ground floor of the large square hall, and the other at the top of the stairs that wound round the peripheral walls to an upper floor of this same hall. The whole atmosphere was feudal, natural and gay without a trace of self-consciousness. All the servants seemed to enter thoroughly into the spirit of the thing as if to show the rest of us what a fine place Switzerland is. Melanie saw I was thoughtful and said, "I know what *you* are thinking about. You are wishing Francesca was here and I have been thinking how she would have enjoyed this". I had no shame in admitting that was exactly what I was thinking about. Oh dear, *how* I wish you had been there! Especially when we walked out into the courtyard again and saw that the colossal tower and keep were now flood-lit. The massive stone stairs, the cobbled court, and this terrific fluted and machicolated tower looked quite magnificent.

It is now past 1.00 a.m. so I must stop. It hardly seems possible that after tomorrow's business meeting it is all over and I set off home to see my dear wife and family again. It seems years since I left you and I long to see you more than I can possibly say.

And now my dear love, goodbye for the present. I don't think I shall really believe I am going to see you till I get back to East Croydon station . . .

1959

St George's Hospital, London[1]

February 3

My darling,
It is visiting hour so I thought I would write, or start to write, a letter. I have at last, stop press, been able to pass a motion. Such a palaver: I must not go to the lavatory; as a special favour I need not use the bed pan, but can have the commode. Why? Because I am so fragile and must not be allowed the slightest exertion. If it is—says probationer but it may be a nurse—what they think it is, I shall have to be cared for in hospital for 5-6 weeks: if it is not, then as far as I could make out, it would be as bad only different. I felt like picking up the pair of them, one in each hand, and putting them both down firmly on the pot. Finally I was not to wipe my bottom but one of them did, or perhaps they both had a turn. I suspect that this thrill was the ultimate aim of a somewhat synthetic panic. There is a fat old woman visitor over the way who has been bursting into the most rich, fruity, bawdy explosions of belly-laugh I have heard for a long time. Perhaps she saw me on the pot. Supper was egg on spinach with some very pale chips: but it tasted quite good. I waved tapioca and treacle away.

The ECG chap showed up and did his stuff. He said it was much the same as this morning and showed nothing particular.[2] The hospital examination routine is very thorough but I suspect it is always a bit rigid. I, who strongly suspect more attention needs to be paid to my digestive upset and old jaundice, noticed that no one asked me about it but I had to draw attention by mentioning the absence of motion. Similarly it was sister who noticed that the graze on my cheek had not been washed as it should have been. But my analytic work convinces me that it takes a long time before people are able to bear a realistic contact with what other people are, rather than with some artefact with which they are familiar.

The HP here said he thought the casualty department had made a mess of it by sending you an alarmist message. I was so pleased to see you I forgot to ask what it was.[3] But it is anyhow so worrying when anyone is in hospital that I am sure if one alarm was not

[1] In spite of an attack of influenza he continued to see patients at Harley Street. On the morning of February 2 he fainted after getting off the train at Victoria Station; an ambulance was called and he was taken to hospital

[2] His ECG had in fact always shown an irregularity which was never satisfactorily explained.

[3] "Your husband has had a heart attack at Victoria Station".

sounded another one would be. Anyway I have *not* got diabetes. And I am feeling very fit indeed now. I feel I ought to set up a huge wail, "Please, please doctor *don't* throw me out of hospital!" on the Brer Rabbit principle. And all the time I wonder how my darling wife is getting on and our babies. For of course they *are* only babies. And you looked so nice and cheerful and loving and beautiful even though I could see the strain and trouble break through. I know it must be so and I wouldn't have it otherwise: you would not be the brave girl I know you are if you were not worried, but I believe if we just try to deal with these things as they come it won't be so bad. Anyhow there is not much else we can do. I must try to find out as much as I possibly can about my physical state and then concentrate on living accordingly. I'm always far too careless—about over-eating particularly.

The old chap next door has just told the young girl House Physician that her examination "tickled" him. There's always a silver lining obviously!

I do hope the children will not be too upset. I wouldn't have them ignorant that hospitals and illnesses exist, but I would like to feel they learn to take them as part of life (one part, not too big I hope unless they are doctors).

I shall *not* send this to you I think. The young chap on my right handed his thick letter for posting to the nurse and the following talk burst on the air.

Nurse: Ooh! It's thick! Lots of nice things in it I expect?

Patient: Yes, *I* know; you'll steam it at the kettle and open it!

Nurse: Pooh! I can do that with my breath.

It's now 9.00 but all the lights are still on so I don't know when they shut down. I suppose we shall all be woken at 5.30 or earlier. Well my dear I must say goodnight for the present. When you come I would like the Braithwaite book on Scientific Method—I put this in in case I forget to mention it. Bless you my sweetheart.

Wednesday morning. Feb. 4th. After a racketty sort of night I feel like unburdening some more to you. The House Physician came round last night and asked after me. He said I should stay in "a few days" even if the ECG was OK. This does not surprise me, but I would like to know how far the "few days" is going to extend. He said my weight was too much and suggested, for my height, twelve stone.

I cannot help thinking, as I read the book I have here on Scientific Method, what a terrible lot of bilge I have read in my time. There has always been a certain amount, too much I think, of gullibility about me, and it makes me swallow a lot of nonsense—not only in books I think—that I could do without. I wish I could feel more confident that I wouldn't add to the flood of rot but of course if I did I would probably lack the necessary self-criticism.

They have been cleaning the walls: that is, brushing the dust off them on to the patients. There have been letters in *The Times* about the dangers of unclean walls and what trade union's job it is to clean them. In fact of course 'the dangers' obvious to bacteriologists and others are just removed from one place to another; at any rate no one is worse off. And over the years the idea probably gets established that it is a good thing to keep clean.

An Irish ward maid has been exchanging a good deal of bawdy with my right hand neighbour who has a photo of his fourth baby which she saw. "No more", was the burden of her lay. "You must have time to sleep sometimes", she told him for the whole of this end of the ward to hear.

I so much wonder how you are getting on. And yet I know that you will be doing everything as usual bravely and cheerfully but with a horrible undercurrent of worry and anxiety which just cannot be helped. And I would so like to help it. I *am* doing what I can: e.g. to take the chance of cutting down my weight which I can do quite easily here because I am in bed and I am not racked by the thought of the delicious treat I am missing. The ward has now settled down to its routine after the cleaners' visitation and I shall have to wait for my ECG.

Later. No ECG. Apparently they think it is too near the old one to be worth doing another—nothing is likely to show. But, and this is bad news, the HP talked about its being a five or six weeks job. And this indeed was a shock. I pass it on as we may as well have our shocks if we have to . . .

This pain in my right side, now I come to think of it, is exactly the same as the one I had to have the X-ray for last year.[1]

February 4

My darling,

It really did seem as if the sunshine had gone out of the ward when you went out just then, but thanks to letters I can start writing straight away. It is a queer thing about love that it teaches you that certain common phrases which seem never to have much meaning

[1] At that time he had cracked two ribs.

are really quite true. If it weren't for you I would not have found that out about the sunshine . . .

Later. Dr Hunter, the chief, has just been in to see me. He ran over me quickly, gave my heart a clean bill and said if my Friday ECG was OK I should be out at the week-end. This has cheered me so much that I keep forgetting I have to have another ECG. And Hunter says he will see me again. I think I *shall* post this straight off to you as I shan't see you tomorrow. Hunter said I ought to take the next week off work. If I could only mobilize some thoughts before I came out I might get a paper done. Unfortunately it is a most complex subject and I don't want to rush into it prematurely. However, I can go on churning and I shan't complain if it is two weeks and not six off work . . .

February 5

My darling,
. . . I begin to feel nervous about the outcome of tomorrow's ECG! Otherwise I feel all right but for the 'catch' in my side when I cough. This remains painful, but I dare say I am becoming too impatient. I am slimming but I am prepared to bet I have lost nothing in weight. I continue to cogitate on my paper[1] but it is a curiously elusive subject and comes and goes. At the moment I am feeling there is nothing in it, but I am used to this . . .

February 6

My darling,
I was so cheered to have your unexpected letter that I nearly wept. I think I must be feeling a lot better as I felt *so* depressed by my breakfast of porridge and hot milk (no sugar) and so wanted to eat the bacon and tomato—but stoically refrained. This is *my* contribution to the treatment and I am feeling more and more that what is the matter with me is the after effect of jaundice ten years ago. I think my liver won't turn all the food into nourishment, but leaves undigested stuff to circulate as poison—hence anything may happen, and it always looks like something else.

. . . Like you I feel only half alive though I hardly realize it till I become wholly alive through your letter. I *must* be pretty alive to lie here being half blown out of bed day and night apparently none the

[1] 'Attacks on Linking', International Journal of Psycho-Analysis, Vol. 40, Parts 5-6, 1959.

worse in spite of the fact that after all I am presumably getting rid of a cold.

I think I feel depressed mostly because I find it difficult to believe I shall get out of here until I am actually back at home. "You have to be difficult to get out of here", says the ward maid. "If you're nice they keep you." I must tell her to spread horrible tales of my 'difficulty'.

And how is my darling wife? You are so brave and look so cheerful and on top of things, and I know you do everything so well that I really wish I could do something worthwhile to match it. And indeed as I write to you I feel I want to be writing a marvellous paper. But if I start on my paper, alas! not marvellous; I feel I don't want to waste time on such rot but should be writing to you.

I could almost write a book on the extraordinary old boy in the corner opposite me. He looks like a scrawny old vulture at death's door but he skips around as merry as a cricket. Some gems of conversation:

Nurse: However many pyjama jackets have you got on?

Patient: Three.

Nurse: It's much too hot for that. (So it is)

Patient: Don't you believe it. I'm not freezing to death for you here.

Nurse: (later) Whatever are you eating?

Patient: Chicken.

Nurse: But you aren't supposed to do that. They are testing you for diabetes. (Looking in the locker) Oh lor! Whatever have you got there?

Patient: Grub. And more chicken.

Nurse: But you didn't ought—

Patient: Never you mind about all that nurse. When I'm at Brighton I never go to the races without a nice bit of chicken and— etc. etc.

He has just been saying that 'they' say the fog is due to cold, but he can't think how they 'do' such things (make the fog perhaps?). He doesn't believe a word of it.

Well, here I lie and feel almost you will have to bring a gun. I feel quite demoralized lying here watching this sort of play go on, feeling perfectly fit, quite comfortable and extremely comfortably off when I know what your anxieties must be. But I must try to get square with my conscience by starting up on some work . . .

February 6

My darling,
As usual when you have left I feel depressed—hardly news of course because what else could I feel? . . .

I know you are having a very bad time and it hurts me that I am not there to help . . . But because you and the family have done something to me I find I spend less time on vain regrets and depressions and fears, and more on an immediate plan than I could have believed possible even a year ago.

February 7

. . . Needless to say Hunter did not turn up nor any of the others: and this means nothing can happen till Monday. The annoying thing is that there are plenty who are ready to *believe* something is seriously wrong even if it is not. And I don't want to give *that* crew any handle, especially with the intense competition for patients that still exists and will become even more intense. That is one reason why I am so anxious to get into print if I can't get into anything else. It is a pity we can't meet to talk—even if you get here there is no chance. But maybe it is easier and better to get one's thoughts into writing.

Later. My dear—it is bad news. I became tired of having no news so this afternoon I asked sister when the ECG would come through. She said it had—and the hope that it was only showing an old lesion has gone. It is a fresh one and I am to lie here and do nothing for myself. I feel more upset than I can say. Of course I knew and you knew that something like this could happen and was a risk when I proposed to you so late in life. The gain was all mine, the penalty, if the gamble didn't come off, was yours. But I hoped something good might come of it for you and now I feel I have let you down. Or rather, that I let you down when I proposed. I should have stayed right away from the Tavi when I knew what was happening. But damn it I would never have done it as I know I am too selfish and really care for no one but myself. But it is not true. And I want you to know how wealthy in happiness you have made me. I really felt as if I had lost it all, but all you have done for me has made me feel rich in happiness—even now, far beyond anything I had imagined happiness was. Bless you my darling girl. My eyes fill with tears whenever I think of the children clubbing together to buy me biscuits; not for unhappiness but happiness: just one of many I should have never known but for you.

I am going to stop now to get on with some work. It is a source of great comfort to me that I am able to do this though it seems without rhyme or reason. It cannot earn me a penny piece or help my dear darling family one jot, which is all I would do if I could, and yet it is somehow a great solace.

This is a very sad letter and I hate to write it to you my *devoted* wife. How much I knew that and yet how happy it made me to see it . . .

There is one consolation: ECG notwithstanding I feel fitter every day and when I *do* stand up—surreptitiously while being put on the commode—I feel very strong on my pins and that in spite of bed and the reducing diet. I would expect to feel pretty giddy and weak.

Now about visits. I think you should put all your priorities into looking after yourself and the children. I am all right here and get the best treatment there is, whatever its shortcomings may be—like all our poor human efforts. So I am safely packed out of harm's way for the time being. I *know* you love me: and that is all I want or need to know. I *know* you are by my side in thought and would be so in fact if it were wise to be here rather than somewhere else. I *know* we must both be troubled and depressed and faint-hearted at times, or we would not be human. I am afraid I have felt like that too often in this letter. But I shall try to be sensible when commonsense shows me you cannot be here . . .

I am wondering whether I ought to take the chance of looking at all that group stuff. I believe it might be very well worth while and it could be the start of a useful piece of work. Or if it is not, then a useful decision to throw the whole lot away.

The time is coming for your visit. I felt so excited I had to go to sleep for a bit and then I thought I shall be so depressed if I miss any of the excitement of your coming and my waiting for you that I couldn't sleep. I just want to say and *do* —I love you . . .

I shall now say goodbye for the present my dearest dear—and start my next letter the moment you are out of the door. The advantage of writing this is that I can think at leisure, and you can read without fear of forgetting or the distraction of no real privacy . . .

February 8

My darling,

. . . I have been re-reading your last letter so as to feel I have something of you which I can actually touch. I am sorry my last letter was so poor—I am not really depressed for long because I usually go over to plans about what can be done about it—whatever 'it' for the time being might be . . .

We had a ten-minute service: half a dozen people filed in including two women. 'Love divine all loves excelling', and then a reading and a prayer 'for the sick and all who minister to them', and 'Abide with me'. Then they filed out. I felt so sorry for them. They were brisk and cheerful and—what else could they *possibly* do? Yet I felt there must be something more or the whole thing is entirely pointless.

I thought how wonderful you looked this afternoon and it makes me feel so proud of you—and myself, though of course I know there is no excuse for that except the best excuse of all— which is you.

February 9th. I had a very good night after I had persuaded them to get rid of two of my three blankets. This morning I have done a bit more writing and checked the reading with it— a quite considerable amount of work though it does not look it on the paper. But I think it is clearly expressed and that is a big problem with this stuff . . .

February 11

My darling,

Here I am—sitting in a chair in a gale of wind. So I am obviously coming on, but what I shall be when the draught is finished is nobody's business . . .

I am at the moment feeling a bit depressed about my paper, wondering if it's all just working round stalking a most majestic mare's nest; a horrid feeling. The fact that there are correlations between scientific hypotheses and interpretations is at first reassuring, but then I begin to wonder if it is only an appearance caused by my saying commonplaces, that everyone knows, in a high falutin' way. Ending up with a blinding flash of the obvious.

I have sent off a note to Parthenope and would like to send Julian and Nicola one. I must try to think of a way I could write Julian a letter he might read for himself and perhaps one he could read Nicola.

February 12. Tea and toast has just turned up but the nurse does not know what I am supposed to have—two slices?—three slices? Marmalade? Me: No, no marmalade and I forget if it's two or three. Nurse: Your egg hasn't come. Do you have an egg? Me: I had one yesterday for breakfast and one for my supper. Nurse: Oh, then it must be an egg. Q.E.D. I suppose, but it hadn't occurred to me that that was how the logic goes. I can see I am getting too well to appreciate all my luxuries here . . .

February 12

My darling,
It was lovely to have you by my side this afternoon. In a way I felt I hardly wanted to talk but was quite contented just to sit there and hold your hand and look at you and hear you talk . . .

Elliott came in this evening for a short time and I asked him about the M.K. Trust meeting. He told me of the progress of the scheme to publish M.K.'s book.[1] But though I was glad to hear negotiations were proceeding successfully I was in fact more concerned to hear about this hare-brained scheme of £70 a year for the support of high grade candidates. He seemed to think it was unlikely to come to much and ended up by suggesting it might just be a matter of having an ad hoc whip round of a limited kind for some special occasion. He also favoured in any case having a standard so high that virtually no one would get a grant . . .

February 13. Another morning, my darling, after a good night's rest. I sometimes feel I ought to have been a recluse, some kind of Oxford don, only then we should not have enough money—we don't have enough apparently anyway, but that is a detail which afflicts anyone who would like to go on Hellenic tours or read good books or go to Glyndebourne. But the serious and disturbing thing is the awful sense of frustration I get because I feel I have something I *must* write but cannot get at it because of the pressure of the stark need to live at all. I can see from my stay here, where it is obvious that sheer force of circumstances makes it impossible to do anything but write and read the appropriate books, how absolutely uninterested I am in anything else except to see and be near you and the family. After that, but really mixed up with the reading and writing, is my work with the patients which I want to do for its own sake. I know I can't shuffle off all these damned financial worries and responsibilities but I certainly feel they are killing my capacity for work—destructive demands for some accursed Trust meeting, group meeting, attendance at a Society meeting, or *anything* almost that will destroy another evening I might have at home. *That* is where I want to be where I can get the rest and refreshment and privacy in which I can think and finally write. Here comes my bloody breakfast I think: it is lucky I am fond of boiled eggs but perhaps it won't be that this time; wet fish perhaps, though I will say that I find most meals appetizing enough. (Later) Boiled egg it was. But four bits of toast instead of three, which makes it two thin rounds. The nurse

[1] *Our Adult World and Other Essays*, William Heinemann Medical Books Ltd., 1963.

today didn't know what I was supposed to have any more than the nurse yesterday, so I feel they must have lost interest in me. If only it would take the form of getting rid of me. Sister has just told me I have a slight temperature which she not unreasonably thinks may be the hangover from my cold. Of course it puts the wind up me and makes me wonder how many extra days of hospital this may mean . . .

(Friday evening) . . . At the moment I am feeling filleted, which makes me wonder—perhaps living on food that has had its 'stuff' removed has the same effect on the person who eats it. The night duty nurse has just come on and tells me she is "absolutely miserable". "So am I", I said, "What are you miserable about?" "Oh, I'm just *fed* up with this hospital and *everything* to do with it." It sounded like extra-sensory perception or projective identification or some such. Anyhow I am in a *bloody bad temper.* And it is a waste of time writing that. But all the time in my heart I have your sweet brave face as it always comes to my mind and as I saw you this afternoon. With your beautiful loving gentle smile. Things will be bad indeed when that cannot make me better. I *am* better, even after such a hell of a dose of medical treatment as Hunter's visit, and there is nothing can have done that but you.

February 14. St Valentine's, and I hope I can produce a better one than this next time. I have been having my lunch at the common table with two others. In fact the ten yards or so there and ten yards back do not at present seem to have done me any harm . . . (The commode has just gone by screaming and whistling on all of its four unoiled castors. It makes me want my oil can.) I wish I felt that they were really certain what is the matter—that is the real point and nothing can matter but to know what the facts are . . .[1]

February 15

. . . I feel momentarily stuck with my paper. It is curious; when this happens I often find I have some other idea, but I am reluctant to pursue it for fear of just leaving a lot of loose ends and never coming to any point. And yet it is also true that taking up the new thread can turn out to have quite an important connection with what I have said before and may indeed be a way round the deadlock . . .

Later. In the upshot I did a lot more thinking but hardly any writing and what there is of it feels as if I had only partially got a grasp

[1] They remained unknown, then and later.

of what I wanted to say. Still, I feel if I have learnt nothing else I have begun to learn that to write something you must write—anything, anyhow, somehow, so long as you write. Only this way is any meaning likely to come of it.

My thoughts are very much with you and the family this fine afternoon. It was a lovely surprise to see you yesterday but it really made my heart go pit-a-pat in a most confusing kind of way; appropriate perhaps to a bashful young man suddenly confronted by a very beautiful girl whom he had been worshipping from afar. Much too much 'afar' for my liking . . .

February 15

My darling,

. . . Last night seemed to be damnably noisy. I don't think I can have been long getting off to sleep but I was awake enough to realize a new patient was very noisy; but this only accentuated my awareness of what a truly noisy hospital this is. Traffic is as far as I know quite incessant at this corner.[1] I don't know why they give me pheno-barb but God knows I would need it to cope with the din. And the row inside seems as bad—steam escaping and what sounds like various forms of machinery grinding away. And it is extraordinary, as another patient remarked some time back, how often someone drops a metal bottle or bed pan with a terrible crash. At the moment (post-breakfast) the whole place is a chaos of Monday morning sweep-up, plus helicopter which has just arrived—this extraordinary mechanical polisher with its wonderful charlady driver. It's no good trying to think.

Later. My darling, Hunter—[2]

[1] Hyde Park Corner.

[2] The letter breaks off here. The consultant had come to say he could go home.

1960

Redcourt

To The Little Cottage, Trimingham, Norfolk March 25

My darling,

It is very nice to have your letter and it made me feel that my hopes that you would have a refreshing and enjoyable break as well as a lot of work might be coming true. I felt as if I *had* had some holiday in Norfolk after I had read it . . .

I have fixed up with Melanie to have supper with her going on from the Gillespie's party: it will do instead of a birthday present. The idea occurred to me this evening and I think must have appealed to her as she cancelled a cinema trip to see me instead. I am of course cursing at the prospect now, but I believe it is the right thing to do and will on balance be helpful. I wish these social events did not quite so often feel like battles in which one always got the worst of it but perhaps it won't be so bad. Anyhow it may help to prevent the propagation of any idea that I am not a proper Kleinian—not a proper anything else either.

. . . I like to have a letter from you as well as telephone and it was very nice to hear you felt it was so lovely. I felt almost I was there when I read about the larks singing . . .

March 27

My darling,

. . . Gillespie was very cordial. I was surrounded by Kleinians. Riviere came, deploring the cessation of the study group and Munro joined the lament. She bubbled away about how well the Clinic went—she got everything she wanted. Personally I can't see how it can be going any differently from usual or what she could be given. On these occasions we are all so warmhearted and friendly, myself included, that it makes me wonder if it is a reaction from a sort of chronic psycho-analytic dislike. But it is there and quite infectious. I began to feel what a good fellow I was too and how popular. S. said *how* much she had liked my paper and *how* true, how *very* true, she had found it. It really quite opened up a new—alley?—vista?—avenue?—it was so very—er, very true. She can't have understood it in fact and I don't know why she should suddenly overwhelm me. However, I told *her* how very—er well, very—er, kind it was of her to—and yes, wasn't it?—quite amazing: I was so glad. But what about God knows. I felt like icebergs.

M.K. apparently became so re-assured that I almost felt I was wasting the price of a meal. I took her to Prunier's which knocked us back £5 and I didn't think it much of a meal either. She pressed on me that she would be *very* glad to discuss my book with me at *any* time and I assured her that of course I would if it really wasn't—really?—well of course I should be delighted. Thirty years ago I might have been, and I think I might then have believed that I am really lovable and valuable and worthwhile, as I would be compelled to think if I believed one third of what I heard last night. And I am just as silly. I squeezed H.'s arm on parting, oh ever so affectionately, and said how much I regretted not being able to do any evening work for the Society but I was hoping to do something during the day for the Clinic. And how was I? Oh marvellous! I looked it, he said. I *am*, I assured him: and how well *he* looked! But maybe I am just tired. However, as I said on the phone, by and large I think it meant I have done myself no harm and probably good. But a paper would not be amiss or they will make it just a bit too like an obituary for me to swallow any of the euphoria.

I rather felt I wanted to get down to a piece of writing to-day. The worst of it is that there were a number of ideas which had clicked into position and I wish I had managed to get them down, but I didn't. As it is, beyond knowing it was to do with 'alpha', I can't remember what they were. And I don't think they always come back.

I find it a bit difficult to visualize what you are doing as of course one very cursory look at the cottage is all I have to go by and at present I cannot see it as anything to do with me. But I shall be glad to see you back and look forward to holding you in my arms: perhaps that's what is missing about the cottage from my point of view.

. . . with all my love and many grateful memories of nine years ago . . .

1964

The Little Cottage

To Wells Rise, London | December 29

My darling,
We are gathered in the lounge. Parthenope is writing, Julian and Nicola reading, and self writing while waiting for the phone to go. The room is beautifully warm because the snow has turned into rain and it is thawing, but it is blowing very hard. The roads have been awful—I fell down twice on the loop road on my way to the village shop, and on the second occasion the rescue team of Parthenope and Nicola likewise fell down. Julian rode his bike and did *not* come off but heaven know why not. Noises very life-like but not at all like Brands Hatch; quite outstandingly moderate in fact.

Our room was so cold I was jolly glad of the electric blanket. Unfortunately my ability to regulate it to maintain an equable temperature is impaired by sleep so I kept on waking up because I was either shivering with cold and stiff as I could well be while maintaining my ability to shiver, or else (having inadvertently switched on to 'high') pouring with sweat and dreaming I was fighting my way through a tropical jungle. I awoke soon after 8.0 but all the others were still fast asleep. So I proceeded to get breakfast and relied on the resulting fracas to wake them, which gradually it did.

I constantly wonder how you are getting on—at this point you rang up. I forgot to ask you if you had the house properly warmed up . . .

December 31

My darling,
. . . It has been a magnificent day and starlit night. Not a cloud in the sky and a keen fresh breeze. I can hardly keep my eyes on the paper for watching the gulls wheeling over the bird table. We put out some Swoop but the time birds take to come back is extraordinary. And even after they do come back they take as long again to wheel around and peer and circle and hover before one dares at last to settle—one toe only and off again; cats on hot bricks could teach them nothing.

The children have all been getting on well. Last night Parthenope was giving Julian a long French lesson on which he seemed to be as keen as she was. They went on at it for over an hour: not my idea of sport but it seemed to go down very well with both parties so who is to worry? Nicola patiently and methodically set about making Origami and did very well with them.[1]

If we get more weather like this we should all be very fit. I wish I could give you what we are having. I find the long sleeps we all have are doing a great deal for us but the person who really needs a rest—you—gets more work then ever. I hope it will seem worth it when you see what you have accomplished.

My work is being done. I have come to the conclusion it is not really a book yet but is more writing for the sake of being able to get the ideas out on the surface. It is painful and heart breaking because there seems nothing to show for it. But I know it's just asking for trouble to think like that—one works to get 'something to show for it' instead of just working; and that is fatal to anything decent.

There is a wonderful sunset—just pure glow of colour, not anything spectacular in the way of clouds — simply radiance. I send it to you with my love. My darling I think of you always. I know what a difficult job you are doing and how trying it must be . . .

[1] The Japanese art of folding paper into intricate designs.

1965

The Little Cottage

To Wells Rise January 1

My darling,

It was a relief to hear your voice when we rang up today in spite of the fact that you obviously have a very bad cold indeed: not surprising since it has had no treatment, or very bad treatment since you caught it. It makes me think I should have stayed with you and let the family come here alone. I might then have relieved you of some of it. But it's no good regretting it now.

I rang up last night as arranged and caught a proper packet of woe from your mother. She seemed to feel all was lost, if one may use so ludicrously cheerful an expression. I felt from her report that there was every chance of your getting pneumonia through sheer neglect of yourself. To make matters worse I knew it would be unlikely that you would tell me much about yourself, except that you were "all right".

At present we plan to come back on Wednesday . . . I hope by then to be able to look after you and to be allowed to do so: I do not want you to slave yourself into such a state that you could not possibly help hating me and all my works. I hope to hear when you ring up tonight that you will at least have no more travelling after today. I assume of course that things have been made as difficult as they could very well be by your being so wretchedly ill you could hardly think.

10 p.m. I had hoped you would ring up before this as it is worrying that you are working so appallingly late. I find it hard to settle to anything when I do not know how things are going with you. Still I should be pretty used to having to think clearly no matter what the distractions may be. I *am* used to it. But I don't feel more skilful at it.

Nor, I imagine, is your job made any more tolerable by the feeling that the move is also the end of our family's first home; still, what can't be cured must be endured.

You have just rung up and you can't imagine what a relief it was to hear you; I even began to imagine you sounded a bit less wretched. It is not that I feel worried about anything—I just feel worried about *everything* and that makes it tiresome and confusing. I do hope you will be able to sleep at Wells Rise tomorrow. I shall feel you have begun to have a home again.

I feel like saying, "Bless you" to Mrs Brockwell,[1] over and over

[1] Our invaluable help for seventeen years.

again, but she would think I must be crazy. It has been a comfort to me to think you had such a stout-hearted person to help.

. . . I think of you and wish you were here to relax in the quiet of this place. Walking in the stiff breeze feels quite marvellous; it feels so austere and pure . . .

August 1

My darling,

. . . We were lucky. It was fine till Newmarket. Then it began to spot. Then it began to rain. By Brandon the heavens opened and it became impossible to see more than 20 yards and soon it cut down to ten yards and going dead slow because it was hard to see a car in front. Goodbye, I thought, to my plans of lunch in the open. Which was very sad because Nicola began to get sick at just past Six Mile Bottom. And of course the poor dears, Parthenope and Julian, made things worse by becoming terribly anxious till I had to cut the discussion very short. With rumblings we proceeded on our nauseating way till within five miles of Swaffham when it began to clear. I shot them all into the church to look at the roof.[1] When they got back some twenty minutes later they had all recovered their equanimity and Nicola had some colour. We went on and some four miles later it was hot and sunny. As I had planned to have lunch at Castle Acre it seemed too good to be true. By Castle Acre not even the roads were wet and we drove into the Priory, took out our lunch and ate it in the precincts in the hot sun, with a cloudless sky and perfect lawns. It was glorious and a good lunch was had by all.

We got to the Cottage by 4.30. There had been a shower or so but mostly brilliant sun. The garden looks very good. I had forgotten the roses would be pretty much in their glory . . .

. . . I hope the builder realizes that it won't be enough to have sound-proof windows in front and a wall that is *not*.[2] It is obvious that the noise in front of the house is going to be drilling more or less indefinitely; they seem to like digging up Wells Rise.

There is some minimal grumble about no TV and therefore nothing to do but join the family for a walk. It makes me wonder if this means there has been too much TV so far. Certainly the air has been less hectic and a bit more peaceful without, but it probably won't last. I detest the lack of inner resource that seems associated with TV and I hope our children haven't gone far on that unpleasant road.[3]

[1] A fifteenth century church with a magnificent hammer-beam roof.
[2] The garage was being converted into a consulting room.
[3] He need not have worried—nineteen years later, two of them have no TV.

I hope all goes well tomorrow and you find some relief and compensation in being without the family as well as the misfortune of not starting your country holiday. The lack of drills almost hits one with a loud clap of silence . . .

August 2

My darling,
. . . We took our things to the beach hut and installed ourselves, but it was an icy swim I can tell you . . . back for gammon lunch with peas (free)[1] and lettuce . . . Then it began to spit and it spat— and spat—and spat till 9.00 pm. Then it rained till 10.00 p.m. Then it poured, drumming on the roof and down the gutters, till we had all gone to bed. This morning I awoke to sun at 6.00 a.m. Glorious! Till 6.15 when it became cloudy. By 7.30 it began to spit. And it spat— and spat — I will tell you the rest later, but that's as far as we have got so far . . .

August 4

My darling,
. . . I've splashed paint about, got on with reading but not any writing. A fine morning and the beach could almost be called crowded. I think the family is *much* better for no television. I am hoping this may mark a turning point. It is such a terribly easy indulgence and completely obscures the existence of other pleasures which are worth far more. Beyond a mild grumble the first day there has been a complete absence of 'gap' in their activities . . .

August 7

My darling,
Yours has just come and I am tremendously cheered to have it. It is nice to hear that things seem to be going well *so far*—how awful to have to qualify one's rapture by 'so fars' and 'up to the presents'!

They have let people in to the strawberry fields at 6d a time because they could not gather them. The field near here is free. Although the whole village had been there the previous day, Parthenope, Julian and Nicola collected 11½ lbs of beauties in an hour!

[1] These were collected from the hedgerows where the pea lorries had brushed on their way to the freezer plant.

I do feel rested despite some horrid anxieties—or is it *because* of them? I never feel at all sure that anxiety is bad for me—I find it often seems to have a good effect. But I *do* miss you terribly even though I am thrilled by the thought of how much you do for me and the children and how wonderful it is to have such a loving and lovely wife. It is almost a compensation that I am always thinking of you . . .

August 8

My darling,
I have just worked it out that it was 47 years ago today that I won the Legion of Honour in the battle of Amiens. One of these useless facts but it reminds me that I wouldn't live my life again if I could help it. Luckily one isn't asked!

For once we have had a bad night due to—of all things—heavy traffic down Middle Street! There has been a continual roar of pea lorries, not only yesterday which we didn't mind, but through the night. The roar, the flash of headlights, and a loud rattling of the window panes in our bedroom—if this went on long or often I wonder if it would affect the fabric of the Cottage.

. . . I wonder how you can possibly get so much crammed into the time before you come down. I am sure you must not extend your stay after Friday or you will get no Norfolk holiday at all . . .

I have not been able to write much but I have done quite a lot of pretty stiff reading. If I could write my two reviews and get them out of the way I would feel happier.

It does make one learn something to do these jobs, but I always feel "Oh, if only I hadn't agreed! How much more time I would have!" But in fact it is only partly true: with me the worst thing is the awful inertia which I seem hardly able to overcome. Yet Money-Kyrle said the other day he could not understand how I managed to get so much work done. So I can't appear to be so frightfully slothful as I always feel. It's queer isn't it? But even *you* talk of never getting anything done. So perhaps it's just a disease—an exaggerated sense of our, or at least my, importance that makes me think I can do so much more . . .

August 9

My darling,
It was lovely to hear your voice especially as I had decided I must not ring you up. I know how you feel about not letting yourself be distracted from the job in hand and I know you do not. It makes me feel very proud of you and rather ashamed of myself. I sometimes think that my trouble is being so pampered by you that I become debilitated by luxuriating in my advantages. But I wouldn't have it any different. And I know it's because of what you do and are that I am a bit better than I would otherwise be.

I felt very proud of our little family today. The Days came about 3 o'clock. Parthenope had made a very good lemon cake. The children just quietly disappeared when I suggested tea and produced two huge plates of assorted sandwiches. ("Take two", said Nicola as she handed them round!). They all joined in the conversation in a lively and not at all obtrusive way. It was very successful and enjoyable. We had it in the garden by the mermaid roses.

It was a superb morning again. We went and bathed at 'our' spot. It really was glorious although the wind has been sharp as it always is. Somehow it doesn't seem to spoil but rather to enhance the swim . . .

I really think the lack of television has been a great advantage. There is no obstruction to realizing the pleasure of home and an early bed when you don't want to play or read any more, and I think it's worth everything else put together for them to learn that life at home can be fun.

A house martin got into our room and couldn't get out. I caught it and showed the children. It was such a pretty creature and hardly seemed frightened. After being admired I tossed him into the air to sail off. It makes one want to know how he got on . . .

August 11

My darling,
I wonder how you are getting on. It is beginning to seem a very long time since I have seen you. And it is I suppose the longest separation from the family that you have experienced since our marriage.

To-day has been another marvellous day. Bright sun in a cloudless sky shining through heat haze carried along by a strong and bracing wind. We bathed at our usual spot. It was wonderful.

There was a chorus of "Happy Birthday to you" over the wall this morning. I must say I think it is a most dreary and repulsive song.

Perhaps I dislike it because one of the facilities offered to the American public is the chance of hiring a special messenger to go and sing the damned thing to the wretch whose birthday is being celebrated. It makes me hot under the collar even to think of it (and even without a collar on, I may say).

I can't go on saying I wonder when we shall see you, so I won't. But we think it. Parthenope hoped you might be getting a little social life to compensate for the hard work. It's a nice idea anyway—and we all acclaimed it. Goodbye my dearest; we all *feel* our love to you so perhaps you feel it too as if it came in gentle waves . . .

August 12

My darling,

Your letter was a great solace to me even though it brought bad news. You cannot come I know till you feel you can come with an easy mind and I thought it would be surprising if you could get away in a fortnight . . .

I cannot get on much with my book because I keep being distracted by wanting to write the article[1] on the Eissler book[2] when I'm trying to write mine and vice versa.

I think we have all got together and know each other a bit better, not least because the children miss you and can realize more how much you do and how much you have to do if you have to be at Wells Rise because of alterations to my consulting room. I am sure they learn a lot by having to clean up, cook etc. I think you'll find them very grown up even if it is a short time. Because a week or so's detached view makes it easier to focus.

And how are you my darling? You really ought to put in a week here in October, doing *nothing* but sleep and rest. And no sooner do I write that than I realize how ridiculous it is to say so and how unlikely you would ever be to do *nothing* even if you could. There is something in it though—I think you will find you can leave it more and more to the good judgment of the children to carry not only more of the responsibility for their own affairs, but also for some of the lighter part of yours . . .

[1] Published in The International Journal of Psycho-Analysis, Vol. XLVII, Part II, 1952.

[2] K. R. Eissler, *Medical Orthodoxy and the Future of Psychoanalysis*, I.U.P., N.Y., 1965.

August 17

My darling,
If I don't write now I shan't have a chance of writing to you because you will be here—another disappointment, but as you say, it's all a matter of perspective!

Of course I am not disappointed at the length of time the job has taken. On the contrary I am amazed that it has been so quick or rather that you have managed apparently to keep them so close to schedule. I know I could not have done it. I just want you to be here and when you are not I feel it; but I would hate it if you felt it a restraint to have had to do so much work for me. I know I shall do better work for feeling that my consulting room is a nice room because it has been made for me by you. And my home. And my family. All made for me by you. It is a sobering thought but is curiously exalting and exciting at the same time . . .

It gives me a wonderful feeling to think I am going to see you soon. It's a sort of mixture of Easter and Christmas and Summer holidays all rolled into one.

The children will be very anxious for you to have a holiday and I think will be seriously hurt and disappointed if you do not make them feel they have been running the house so well that they may as well go on with the good work. So shall *I*.

. . .I can't make up my mind whether I shall be so disappointed if you can't come tomorrow that I won't be able to stand it, or whether it will be so exciting having another day of expecting you that I can't bear to miss it. I wish you could hear the church bells ringing. They must be ringing in my heart I think.

Goodbye my dearest, for the *present* (it only lasts a moment this time!)

1967

The Little Cottage

To Wells Rise July 29

My darling,

The journey down was so awful for Nicola that the only thing to do is to tell her now that she and Julian will go home by train; otherwise she cannot but dread it. No sooner had I diverged to go by Ely, in the hope that all would be well, than she started again and even a short stop in Cambridge, another for breakfast outside Ely, a long one this, another in Ely to go over the Cathedral and quite a walk around as well, made no difference. She was really ill all the time: and of course she kept apologizing for the stops although I kept telling her it did not matter in the least except that she was having a rotten time. Of course the journey was very slow so we didn't get in till about 2.30. We all went and had a bathe then.

. . . I suppose it is a sign of age, but I would like our children to marry and live happily ever afterwards. I gather it just does not happen. Whether it is the private affair, or international, from Rhodesia to Vietnam, Russia to Mao Tsetung, nothing seems to go right ever; extraordinary isn't it? And if it does go right one suspects it is only for some people and they are just beastly. What are psycho-analysts supposed to cure? I really do wonder.

I am beginning to feel restive and that it is time I had some 'thoughts', but I realize it is only the third day of the holiday. It's a bore your not being here . . .

In the course of my gloomy feelings I could not help thinking what the original Pilgrim Fathers must have felt like when *they* set out for America.[1] At first it seems a bit far fetched, to say the least, but I am not so sure that it is. I *do* regret leaving England; I do feel anything but confident about the kind of reception one will get there. Yet I am not sure that the stories told us are quite as easily explained as people think. There *is* much pessimism in the U.S. about psycho-analysis: there *ought* to be more pessimism about it here. But I feel doubtful about what can be done, not least by myself, either here or in the U.S. What else *can* one feel? And how is it to be put to the test except by going? . . .

[1] *We* set out on January 25, 1968.

August 2

My darling,

. . . I certainly think that the Cottage has done its job for the children as until to-day you could not have had more favourable conditions and yet 'boredom' has never been far away. Of course one might argue that it is because we are leaving, but I think it would be worse if we weren't.

. . . My mind has been running a lot on leaving this country. It is extraordinary how mixed my feelings are. I feel I should be very sad, and sometimes I am when I hear the thrush or the blackbird singing and expect to miss them. But though people warn one about the treachery and so on of Americans, I feel people are very much alike and that there are qualities of people here which are just as nasty (even one's own!). I hope we can get a chance to talk freely. Yet it is difficult to know what we can say that we have not already been over . . .

To Los Angeles — October 3

My darling,

It already seems years since you went and this place is a bit desolate in consequence. I hope you are having a good journey. I am churning over the paper and feeling jolly glad I shan't have to give more. Wednesday. The 'paper'[1] (of course I didn't read it) went off all right. At first I thought no one was coming—only one or two there five minutes before the start. But it filled up. They all stayed (except about three) till past the end and there was no hostile demonstration.

. . . Your letter has just come in. I am so relieved and glad to have it. You must have been very tired and it is lovely of you to have written to me at once. I felt a bit as I did in the First World War — I couldn't bear to write home because I felt I couldn't *think* of home. But I was only nineteen then and there was some excuse. I too wish I was with you; it is awful to think you have to do all this load of business by yourself,[2] and I know you must feel it a wretched responsibility to meet all the snags which are sure to crop up without a chance of talking it over. *You* have not a moment too much time—*I* feel it is an age to have to wait another fortnight.

[1] 'Negative Capability', unpublished, but see *Attention and Interpretation*, Chapter 13. Tavistock Publications, London, 1970.

[2] House-hunting.

Julian rang up—he said he had nearly scored twice in rugger but each time the full back had got him. He seemed to think this very unreasonable! I remember the feeling myself.

I thought the 'paper' went well. Of course I spoke direct; too many 'ers' I think, but I haven't spoken for a long time and I did not, as you know, relish the circumstances. I think I spoke to the point and a number of people seemed to feel that *this* time a lot more people grasped the general idea. It might have turned out anyhow—including a boycott. There is no doubt that the Klein Group has been very upset but I think they needed it. But there must have been about 130 people which is as much as anyone has a right to expect. Furthermore there was no nonsense about my going (tears of grief etc.). Just a straight forward exposition by me of my ideas about how things should go and how I at least tried to make that happen. I think the fact that it was straight forward talk, 'to be continued in our next', all helped. And as I say, they stayed to the end.

I do hope you will not feel you are landed with an impossible job. I know what a terribly difficult one you have and I am sure you realize I shall do my best to fit in with such plans as you can make. Do please try to get in some rest and relaxation. It is too heavy a job for one person to tackle without some time in which to dismiss the whole job from your mind. Even in your kind of work I think you need to dismiss 'memory and desire' so as to have as clear a mind as possible for the decisions. You can only do 'the best you can'—not 'the best'. But I know you don't need to be told this.

. . . Heaven knows where anyone is safe or reasonably secure with the U.S. so shaken by Vietnam. And this country seems unlikely to get into the Common Market with the recent EEC report that we are bankrupt. Why *should* a successful Europe want a bankrupt Britain which has also a labour force completely out of hand and strike-riven? . . .

October 7

My darling,

. . . I had my first sitting with Ishbel,[1] about an hour and a quarter, which was quite cramping, and as I was kept talking on psychoanalysis I was quite exhausted by the end. She seemed to prefer that I should not look, so I did not and do not know what it is like.

. . . As I have no reason for writing this except to say "I love you",

[1] Ishbel McWhirter, the painter.

and I can't just keep putting that, I have a minor problem! Julian is sitting reading *The Battlefield* —the William Mayne you wanted me to get. I have also given him a Trollope to take back, *The Way We Live Now*. He was surprised to see on our London map that Anthony Trollope was at Harrow so that persuaded him to try in spite of his feelings of distaste for the Barchester books. It is very pleasant to hear him playing the piano. He plays extremely sensitively which is so unlike most boys I am used to: it really is a pleasure and it makes me feel I am at home for the first time since last Tuesday. I could hardly believe that days could drag so much . . .

October 8

My darling,
Julian has gone off so I am starting again. It might seem rather desolate again now he has gone, but I do feel we are not so far from each other in spirit and that is curiously comforting . . .

Your darling letter arrived this morning. I am glad you do not feel disillusioned on second acquaintance but rather confirmed in your feelings about living in California. It is good that both houses turn out to have possibilities. Of course I know our friends are delighted to see you: I shall do my best to contain my jealousy within reasonable bounds; I hate jealous and envious people — they are such a bore . . .

October 10

My darling,
. . . I have just shown a very nice woman over the house and she is so taken with it that she's bringing her husband to look at it at 2.30 on Saturday. Now *I* shall have to say that I don't know what my dragon of a wife will want but alas, much as I would love to give it them on a plate, I can't because it is my wife's house! I don't think I fill the bill as a very exacting financial husband . . .

October 11

My darling,
I hope that your very next letter will say you have had some letters from me. I think your trip is *quite* anxious enough for anyone, even

if things went through without a hitch; it is intolerable that you should have the feelings of loneliness too, simply because I was too stupid to send you a note right from the first. I know how your love and support sustain *me* in this job and make anxieties easy to bear. I think our decision to leave has stirred up quite a bit here in our colleagues. I answered queries in the (extended) Klein group tonight. It was clear that they were jolly glad to get it and I think they were again very much impressed. Indeed I do feel that what I have been saying is requiring a new orientation in all practising analysts . . .

October 14

My darling,
What very good news and what a relief it must be for you after all your efforts and horrible anxiety! Thank God you have the courage to do things I cannot and could not manage; though to be fair to myself I think I have a kind of courage though it does not feel like it . . . I hope you felt you *really* like the house and felt it was something you wanted. I know I said I regarded the work as paramount, and of course I do, but I think it essential you should feel it could be *your* home as you get to know it. The trouble here is that this is a wonderful consulting set up but it is only a home because *you* live here, and while you live here. I hope, my sweetheart, that you feel proud and happy though I know there is much more to do—it is only a beginning. But such an important one.

I am just back from Ishbel's—I saw the portrait. I think I am in rather a tense position. She said she had made me rougher—had not put in my benign look but more the tension of when I am talking about work. Personally I think she is too polite to say, as *I* think, that it shows my bad temper. I don't think you would like it but she says she will show it to you when you return and you can judge for yourself.

. . . I am surprised to find how indifferent, except for occasional pangs, I feel about leaving England. It is sad to feel one is *not* sad. Once I would have thought it impossible to leave one's country and one's friends, but somehow things change so much that it is not so. Still I think it must be because one's whole attitude has altered . . .

October 16

My darling,
. . . Tonight there is news of terrific fires—burning near Los Angeles. Of course I get fed up: and wish you were here. This letter I shall send off but I fear it will not get to you before you leave. As long as you are here safe I don't mind. It is a howling gale and raining too—great gusts against our windows. I wish you could have the rain for your fires . . .

The impudent violence of unofficial strikers is only matched by the feebleness of our legally constituted government. One fears the conservatives would be feebler still if possible.

Today I thought the days were deliberately crawling. It's no use the time coming nearer for your return if each day lasts a week!

It's blowing harder than ever and I must stop and go to bed. With all my love my darling. How I long to see you. And what is the good of saying that? I don't know. And the wind sounds as if it is from the west so perhaps it won't delay the plane! It *sounds* as if no plane would take off in such weather . . .

It's a pity I can't tell you exciting things about what I am doing because I seem to have either no news at all, or fears that we are on the verge of a disastrous lawsuit.

October 18

My darling,
It is a *glorious* day, sunny, cold fresh wind, brilliant blue sky. I am writing this in the 'tea interval'. Appropriately the hooter has gone on the building site. They seem to have an enormous number of tea intervals—a reform which people like us have long advocated as leading to more efficiency. Rail strikes, dock strikes, etc. etc. seem to be the result, but I am not certain that in the end it will not lead to great advances and indeed may already be one. It is a pity that we are so weak though.

And I wonder how my darling is? I feel as nervous as a cat waiting for you to come. I dare not count the hours and cannot keep from doing it. So if you are reading this before I see you please remember I'm in a highly nervous state. I don't think I can have been in love before. Believe me it's *awful* and lovely at the same time . . .

The news tonight is as bad as it could be. We shall be lucky if we get through without revolution—that is if *this* is not it *now*. Gunter[1] hauls out the old chestnuts about Communists—I suppose it's the best they can do.

[1] Ray Gunter, Minister of Labour.

1968

En route to Buenos Aires

To Los Angeles July 28

Darling,

I am starting this on the plane, presumably nearing Buenos Aires. It is a marvellous sunny morning even on ground level as far as one can see from 35,000 feet. After leaving you to board the plane we took off not too late—I hope you and the family did not wait. I slept most of the time but the scenery was too wonderful to miss for the first hour and a bit. I woke up, more or less, to hear the plane would be late, but consoled myself there was plenty of time and I would as soon pass it stuffing food on the plane as hanging about the deserts of corridors. I began to be a bit nervous when I realized it was 7.0 p.m. We were reassured when the captain said all services were delayed so that those with connections need not worry. Having reached Kennedy Airport, dark and visibility nil, we circled it for an hour and half. At 8.45 we landed.

I rushed madly off. Not a soul to ask but a chaos of public. At the exit I found the first Pan Am official who told me to catch the bus—not to worry about baggage as it was booked through. At the entrance I waited, then saw a bus labelled Pan Am—the only inconspicuous label I've seen in the U.S. Driver said "Jump in". Finally I got to a desk—interminable conversation between official and elderly woman. "Go to Gate 6." Told we could embark at 9.30. "For Buenos Aires?" "Have you got a ticket?" I showed it but he had lost interest. Afterwards I could see his point. The crowds were terrific and it was very hot and noisy. "Only one small bag each allowed." People turned back right, left and centre. Luckily it was all I had. At 9.45 we were allowed on and I got my seat, having decided there was nothing to be done about luggage. At 10.0 the captain announced that he was sorry for the delay but—10.10 just off when the weather report from Caracas came. 10.35 just off, when we had taken on extra fuel. 10.45 no report of weather from Rio but would be off at once. 11.15 the flight plan had not come through but we—yes, you've guessed it—we were off. 11.30 we began to move. 11.31 stopped. 12.0 moved to runway. 12.10 captain announced that since eight other craft had to get off we would be delayed 20 minutes—very sorry. 12.45 started rushing down runway. Airborne! Dinner would be served. I had hors d'oeuvre and skipped the rest to a small piece of cheese—Maxim's of Paris and 'ever so gay'. It is now 10.0 a.m.

and we are crossing a huge river. No one knows or cares what. Some towns are appearing. Their names must be military secrets I think. We seem to be descending so I had better stop.

Believe it or not, we *did* descend and all in one piece. Grinberg came on to the tarmac and ushered me through— VIP treatment. My case was there and was passed first by customs without examination. Grinberg fetched the car and we set off. I was feeling very hot and dirty and unshaven.

They say they have no racial problem because there is no indigenous Indian race as in the other countries—'Stout Cortez' having been particularly firm and modern in his outlook, I imagine, and leaving no doubts about who was to be 'stout' if anyone. They assured me that the weather—brilliant hot sun—was quite atypical; it *always* rains! We passed the estuary of the River Plate. It looked very fine but you could not see the other side.

Tonight, 6.30, Grinberg is to take me to the Cattle Fair—*the* one in the world—and to dine before an early bed. Up here in my room I found a basket of chocolates, white with blue flowers, all made of sugar. *Not* slimming. It reminded me, if being perpetually reminded were necessary, that you should be here. I have an idea which makes me think you had better come here and talk to some of these people anyhow, but of this more later.

Two maids have been and, as far as I can tell, have sealed the place up hermetically. The people in the streets don't look at all well-to-do but perhaps this is the Sunday milling crowd of flotsam and jetsam. I am not feeling quite so *jet*sam myself since I had a shower.

Later. I have just finished the day's work and am on the verge of going out with Grinberg. I have managed my eight hours without undue fatigue—indeed I think I was less exhausted than quite a part of the audience. But then they had to listen to *me* and I did not.

Last night they took me to the barbecue (indoors, although the weather yesterday and today has been marvellous—they all argue it should be humid and raining) and there they stuffed me full of barbecued meat till I thought I would burst. No ill effects so far but I don't know what they are going to do tonight.

Give everyone a kiss from me. And keep very special ones for yourself. Remember I love you always. Tell the children I will write as soon as ever I can and give Julian my special love for his birthday. I hope it will be one of 366 very special days in the year.

With all my love my darling. I *miss* you . . .

July 30

My darling,
. . . Last night my lecture—about 300 people smoking and jammed tight—ended at 11.15 but I was still functioning though I had worn out two translators. So perhaps it has been a success from the *work* point of view.

. . . C. has shown up and introduced herself as my admirer. She invited me to the home for "a really simple, quiet, restful time", for which I thanked her but sidled out oozing gratitude at every pore. After the evening lecture she announced that she had all the symptoms I had been talking about. I am sure she is right, poor thing, but she has certainly left out all the important symptoms. Unfortunately there are seven more working days to go and if she has not changed to bitter hatred at being rejected before many hours have passed I shall be extremely surprised. Quiet restful home—mon pied! as we say in France . . .

August 2

My darling,
This is 7.30 on Saturday evening and I am feeling a bit loose in the mental joints and as if it were Sunday as well. Perhaps it is a sign of mental loosening that I throw back to depressing feelings that it is Sunday at the old prep school at Bishops Stortford: how penetrating these memories are! I did *not* write to you on Thursday or Friday because I had not the time to do more than write to the children on Thursday, and yesterday evening I went to a party at Dr Mom's house—he is the President of the Society—to meet the training committee. I thought the evening was passing quite well, that is that I might get to bed by midnight, when they announced amidst great enthusiasm a cabaret show in my honour. It turned out to be five men, all brothers, and a girl, unrelated. I did curse it that we had not, or I had not, agreed to a five week tour of Latin America for the whole family, but no doubt it is better as it is. I must say I am a bit surprised to find I do not know a damn thing about Latin American, or indeed American, geography. I had not realized that the next stop is Patagonia. Anyway, the members were all introduced to the celebrated Dr Bion. They were all people who had been to university—a qualified doctor, a dentist, a biologist and so on—but they had never practised but had gone straight into show business after fulfilling their promise to their father to qualify first. I *cursed* bitterly to think you were all in Los Angeles when you might have been with me.

I was shown the instruments which were to be used: a primitive drum, pre-Colombian flutes, a sort of banjo the back of which was the skin of an iguana, and a pretty conventional guitar. They were dressed, except the girl who was in blue, in very handsome gaucho costume, jet black, buttoned up jacket, black 'wellington' boots and a very striking deep red scarf-shawl affair. The dancing and singing were, to my eye and ear, pretty usual folk lore though with great verve and in a pervading spirit of good humour and kindliness. I was placed in a kind of throne—the Royal Box—which I tried to occupy with proper dignity. Alas, I thought, if *only* you and the family were here! (I won't say this any more.) At one point a young psycho-analyst's wife took the place of the girl and, having learned these dances at school and university, performed with great vigour with the drummer who took the floor for the dance. (They could all change instruments at will and play the other one's speciality.) Finally I was presented with a long-playing record of theirs, on the illustrated sleeve of which they had written their autographs. After shaking hands with each in, I hope, a truly 'noble', if not royal manner, we finished. Home by 2 a.m. after eight hours of work.

Today I was taken to the Grinberg's country house at Escobar, near the Parana River thirty miles away; lunch after elevenses; journey back here by 6.30, so I don't think I've done badly especially as on the journey there three analysts talked to me very loudly and very insistently about the Oedipus Complex and particularly to the effect that the father starts the trouble by trying to kill the children. I just felt O Gawd, O Gawd, what have I done? But I either woke up or things began to get better. It was a gloomy dark day—dark cloud as in London but not cold. The country was as flat as a pancake—the pampas— but not unattractive to eyes that were not used to it. I'm having supper at the moment; an English couple, in which the man is loud voiced, are two tables away. He talks with great aplomb about "bloody waiters", thus showing the superiority of the FLAG to these bloody dagos. Funny, it only makes me feel inferior. Most of these chaps know English anyway.

. . . People have come to hear my lectures, seminars and supervisions from Brazil, Venezuela and Uruguay. As Grinberg says, they are nice people. And I must say I think he is quite right. They have also been very generous in their appreciation.

. . . This will I think be the last letter because it will be quicker to bring the next one. I love you. I am sustained by the thought of you . . .

Sunday morning. As the post does not go yet I may as well add a few lines. It is a lovely sunny morning but I have refused an invitation for lunch as I feel I could do with a bit of my own company so as to have a bit of yours—in thought at least. As time goes on one realizes that the reception as a sort of 'great man' is very seductive and makes it the ideal approach to one's weak spots—the true situation reveals itself in time and it becomes clear that they want you—if they find they cannot do without you. And I do not doubt that is the situation here just as much as in Los Angeles. Looking back on it now and assuming one could find it out by some other means, the idea would be to have found and stuck to a nice home (ideal) in a nice England (ideal too) and paid three-weekly trips to such foreign parts that wanted one. Even so the idea is a false one of skimming the cream (or cash!) off life and leaving the old rubbish to someone else. An idea as old as the hills and much more ephemeral . . .

August 6

My darling,

. . . On coming back to the hotel I found your first letter. And I know how you felt because by Sunday evening I was sure I would *never* last the time. However, the work has been a relief. Very 'enthusiastic' reception and although I think I now know better than to allow myself to be taken in by it, it is a comfort and a nice change after Los Angeles analytic 'enthusiasm'. However, I am quite sure that the astringent atmosphere of Los Angeles is better for *me*—if we can stand it. I hate to think of the time you are having and the anxiety *you* have to put up with. I am glad to hear of the family and that you think they are having the holiday they need. In a peculiar way I feel I am having the *work* I need. Something was going wrong in the work in England—not only mine. I can't, as you know, pretend I like it, but there it is. I *like* the people here, but it is bad, as I have learnt to our cost, to allow one's self to be seduced. I have therefore been careful to accept the minimum of invitations on the excuse of 'need to keep fresh' and 'work'. In fact I have put in a terrific amount of sleep during the day and consequently have slept at night. The arrangement of ¼-hour breaks between hour sessions works very well. I even manage to have coffee *and* go to sleep in that time.

. . . I think the fine weather *did* come here. They all agree it has been an exceptional winter. The one or two dark and gloomy days have had the effect of recalling what I do not like about London and England. Still, I would not have our children grow up in the L.A.

atmosphere. Drugs for all on tap from ten onwards and no other inner resources is just not good enough.

In another minute or two I must go to my seminar lecture and I feel I have not an idea in my head. Now for a think, or I shall stand there with my eyes popping out of my head and jaws moving but *no sounds* coming out.

Thursday—only. It sounds terribly unappreciative. The time has resumed its slow pace which it had the first days and now I feel as if I shall not get through the last three hours of today, let alone the whole of tomorrow and the whole of Saturday before I see you. And the horrible feeling that I do not know what the Yanks will get up to. I feel like an old goose who eyes the human kind with suspicion as much as to say, "Now I wonder what devilment you are planning" . . .

Later. Well, I have got through Thursday—not I think so badly as I feared. I have the confidence to believe I can do it and then begin to get anxious about the confidence. They have recorded every blessed seminar and lecture and are going to let me have a copy.

And now for the last eight hours! . . .

1969

Los Angeles

To London May 30

My darling,
It seemed very queer to come back to an empty house but nice to see the message in red on the blotter. And the table set! I find I tend a bit to wander round and give a shout to you to look at a bird or some similar irrelevance. If I have a dazed bachelor look when you come back do not be too surprised. I have been doing, and expect to continue doing, some very hard thinking about these extraordinary people and the extraordinary situation here. One glance at a daily newspaper would convince anyone that it goes far beyond any office. I do not know where or how to tackle it. Today talks of: Stravinsky going to leave L.A. because only two of his works have been performed; San Francesco and L.A. dangers of earthquake; the Dean of U.C.L.A. visiting hunger-strikers outside Royce Hall and congratulating and encouraging them on their strike to get National Guard off the campus; Federal Government subpoena-ing various authorities of various California universities to produce lists of students with grants who have taken part in disorders. Now—what do I do? Go and psycho-analyse someone? Someone in this country must respect the truth for them to be able to put spacecraft round the moon. I am sorry to write such a horrible 'letter'. It is so much in my mind—and it so much concerns us both—that I can't think of anything else, other than the constant thoughts about you and the children, and they are hardly news (the thoughts I mean). Still, here they are—I love you, and the children—in parallel so to speak . . .

May 31

My darling,
. . . I wish I could tell whether I am just paranoid or whether I am right in thinking that there is a very careful discrimination against English gentiles. But I don't think an analyst doing analysis is welcome—he shouldn't be. Anyway, *who* is welcome? I remember the great enthusiasm for Belgian refugees in 1914-15. I remember how unpopular they became. I remember how fed up *they* became as the British were not as hospitable or appreciative as they should be. Everyone expects to be loved and wanted and especially I think by

the 'new boy'. Everyone expects the new boy to be loving and lovable. The thing is to have a clear view and, for us in particular, whether we can survive in this or any other place . . .

June 3

My darling,
I have been reading an article on Britain's finances. The writer had the idea that everything is marvellous and it is hard to see what anyone is worked up about. Optimistic or pessimistic, one feels they are all pure phantasy and yet there must be a fact buried somewhere.

I have been trying to sort out my psycho-analytic ideas. It is pretty well a whole time job in itself but luckily practice is an aid not a hindrance. I have one great advantage over most: I do at least realize the importance of evidence or, to put it another way, observation, which brings me back to the present, the wretched business of really not being able to know what is going on with one's family.

It already seems as if you had been away for years but that is the fault of its being a long week-end at the start. I expect to have some patient sessions vacant in the coming fourteen days. One has all one's old familiar anxieties re-juvenated! . . .

June 4

My darling,
. . . I had better send you all my love today if it is going to get to you in time for our anniversary. It is incredible—we would never have guessed the facts if we had tried on that June day since which so much has happened. The time here seems to crawl and go too fast as the same time. I feel almost as if I have been a bachelor here all my life and can hardly remember when you were here, and as for thinking back to our marriage, it is almost as if I dreamt it. And now it's another whole week till I see you again. It will take me another week (perhaps!) to get thawed out again . . .

June 6

My darling,
I hoped I would have a letter from you today yet it was a great relief when I found it in the box. I thought I would begin to feel 'it is only one more week', since it is Thursday, but not a bit of it. Instead of that I have been feeling that I could *never* get through another week.

In fact things have really gone not at all badly. I gave X. a session which was one long ultimatum on Monday, feeling sick at heart after it because I felt I did not want to lose a patient. He turned up again on Tuesday though; more ultimatopoeic (if you grasp my meaning) sessions, that and the next day, together with a phone call from Mrs X. asking what to do and whining fit to burst about her 'assuming I would tell the boy what to do'. "Suppose he says he won't come?" "Tell him you will give him a lift." "But I find I can't carry him if he won't—". Stifling a "Good God!" I suggested she might tell him to go but leave him to get on. If she cannot see that people in a home *all* have to sacrifice some liberty if life is to be tolerable, one wonders how any boy could have a hope of progress or disciplined growth . . .

June 8

My darling,

Your letter was very welcome and a great consolation. I wonder how many, if any, psycho-analysts know that a wife or a husband is essential to any decent work. I do not think it appears in the literature except by implication. Melanie didn't *say* so, but I expect that she did not in fact think so unless it was latterly.

So it is the eve of our anniversary. I think it is quite extraordinary the course our lives have taken, as far as it very well could be from the conventional run . . .

J. says I ought to take out an 'Errors and Omissions' insurance. He says that otherwise anyone feeling hostile can claim damages and even if they failed to get costs the legal expenses of defense alone might be very great. Of course this has been one of my nightmares and I have no idea what one can do about it. Analyse it? That is the answer, but how this is to cope with a wealthy delinquent like Mrs X. I don't know. Even assuming one can get an insurance—a large assumption as I am not 'a doctor'—one wonders how much use this is and how much it is pure phantasy . . .

9th June. La voici l'heureuse journée. I love you; but it is a long time to go to June 12th. I am feeling homesick on behalf of the children and you who have to lose each other.

10th June. . . . A. is in a bit of a spin because when talking to a fellow member at the tennis club he chanced to mention, in conventional reply to his acquaintance's report that he had injured his ankle, that he, A., uses a cold compress and that it is very successful. On Saturday he was told that the acquaintance was suing him for damages for wrongful diagnosis and negligent treatment! So it is *not* just me. On the other hand it is not just NOT-ME either! . . .

Amherst College

To Los Angeles August 21

My darling,

. . . As far as planning went the whole exercise could hardly have gone more smoothly. To start off with, all *your* planning had only one major defect—that you were not there and the conference was. The rest of it was a much more mixed business and even so that was really what it was there for—to be a mixed business.

. . . Ken Rice, looking white haired and older, was the same as ever. It soon became evident that R.S. was very nervous, as this was his first experience as Director of the Conference. He was scared stiff of A.K.R. and self, though I did not get wise to this or its extent quick enough or I would have tried to keep my mouth shut. I don't think I would have been successful as he was also continually trying to make me talk and express my views which he then did not like—either because I expressed different ones or because he thought, rightly, that I was trying to re-assure him.

The next morning—the members were to arrive by 4.0 p.m. for tea and Opening Meeting at 4.30—was passed in continued Staff discussion and this took much the same form. After the plenary I was so unfortunate as to be talking when the meeting ended and the Staff walked out. I had not realized that according to the real rules of Groups—as laid down by Ken—he insisted on split second termination of each meeting, and by the time I had finished my sentence the Staff had disappeared round the corner and I couldn't find where they had gone. So I went to my room. K. turned up about 20 minutes later and said there was 'consternation' about my disappearance. I thought he was joking, but at the final meeting of Staff I discovered to my amazement that he had understated the facts. R.S. held forth on how 'everybody' had wondered where I was. 'Everybody' likewise, according to R.S., talked of nothing but me and 'one' person had said how I stayed behind and had an adoring crowd at my feet. Luckily it did not occur to me to mention how like the Infant Jesus holding forth in the synagogue—'and they were astonished at his teaching'—or I might have been tempted to say I hoped he had not been taking counsel with the Elders as to what to do with me (then the fat *would* had been in the fire). It ended up with my being very depressed and inclined to pack my traps and clear out. However, I thought of Shaw's advice, 'Never resign: get kicked out', and decided on the latter. But the continual 'Bion—Bion—Bion—' did ultimately make me a bit angry and impatient. All praise—'of course'. Apparently R.S. had been subjected to some criticism—how much I don't know—because of his change of plan by which I was not taking the Study Group as originally arranged, and in fact, though it was to some extent to my advantage, I was practically cut off from any close contact except in large groups where there were always Margaret Rioch and himself present. Further it became clear to me that while no one was supposed to be able to know, *I* was to express my views to the Staff and act as—private chaplain? physician?—to R.S., and only on the last day and a half to have a group of six, not twelve, to myself. In fact as I say, as I do not know this 'culture' I was very lucky and I think got some insight into what goes on here. And not very comforting insight it was either.

They had a ridiculous 'sit in strike', almost obligatory I gather, as an expression of the way to behave in groups. I suspect it's a lack of interpretation, but it is not clear to me what interpretation it is supposed to be or what the unfortunate R.S. was supposed to do. I did have the consolation that I did not have to deal with it and that this kind of behaviour is not reserved merely for foreign gentiles. In fact the effect it had on me was to have greater sympathy with and respect for R.S. Details I shall have to give you by degrees and in person. Nice thought. And when you read this you will be here! All my love my dearest . . .

1972

Los Angeles

To London July 11

My darling,
. . . I was with the doctor about 40 minutes—mostly chat but some chest listening. The verdict was—'Fine: heart OK; BP ditto; weight ditto; lose a bit more to have a margin. Exercise: walk; swim; and cycle though obviously *not* uphill (which I would never have dreamt of doing at any time in my life even when I was playing first class rugger for Oxford).

. . . Mrs Y. turned up at the hour which she had cancelled, swearing she had not. I would not see her. I shall end up by being condemned to have a spine of my own—let's hope. It would at least be something. If so, this place will earn my gratitude for doing something for me which the whole of my life has failed to do. A bit late perhaps . . .

July 12

7.25 p.m. . . . Answered a call from B. and declined an invitation thus no doubt causing umbrage. Next week then? No, not really. Trout are marvellous! Mmm—but no. Will call on Tuesday. Out. Thursday then? Out. Friday? Perhaps; packing. My God, my God. Don't people *love* me! Naturally I am filled with admiration for myself. Aren't you jealous? And envious? Don't you wish you were loved too? But I am getting too old, tired and unappreciative. Do you think it possible that Greta Garbo spoke the truth when she said she 'wanted to be alone'?

July 14

9.45 p.m. It seems terribly late but not surprising as after I got back here I walked to the bank, went into the market, found they had cherries which I had hoped for but was surprised to see. And, carrying a sale price Jerusalem Bible walked back. I knew Julian had been interested in the Dali Jerusalem Bible and that dismissed the last vestige of my common sense and conscience. The paperback is $9 and as this was $19 you can see I hardly put up a resistance.

On the way back in the taxi, the driver regaled me with an account of his day's frustrations. One story was of how a woman had a ball thrown full in her face because she had asked the boys to play a little further away. It smashed her glasses. She rang up the boy's mother who said she could do nothing because she had no money and lived in penury as her husband had left her. So she got her lawyer son to ring up. He said she had no redress in law but he would try. Same result, but the mother said it was not *her* boy who had done it and suggested calling the mother of the friend. This, with some misgivings, he did and found he was talking to a colleague. He referred him back to the first woman. So he explained the tragic circumstances of the first woman who couldn't possibly re-imburse his mother for the glasses. The lawyer laughed incredulously and explained it was typical. "In fact", said he, "she is as rich as Croesus. She lives in a $240,000 house in" (naming a very wealthy and luxurious place just near UCLA), and that her husband was also v. well-to-do, and that they lived on the best of terms. The taxi driver's woman friend, who is *really* poor, at this point felt it was time to call it a day. The driver said, "You can't cope with the rich". "That", I said, "is why they are rich". But I made a somewhat rueful note to myself that this could very well be Mrs J.—whose addiction to the truth is outstanding and whom I am supposed to be analysing but who has completely shot the analysis to bits.

One more example of serendipity? The driver may have been sent to drive me so as to tell me the cautionary tale. Angelic intervention? I think it must be so . . .

July 15

. . . I was a bit surprised to find how much I had the feeling you were still in the house—still have!—mostly when I am not quite awake, but otherwise also. I hope my 'spiritual' self has not been too greedy and obtrusive, nor interfered with your current pleasures . . .

July 16

. . . I am worried at the prospect of my interview with Mrs Y. tomorrow—I didn't see her last week because I took her at her word and *did* give her session to someone else. Naturally she pursued her course of making a damned muddle by turning up and saying she had *not* cancelled. When I said I could not change the Monday, she said, "Let's leave it". Of course ambiguous, and could mean leave it that she *was* coming. This kind of expression of hostility by shooting the analysis to bits and then running the analyst is a very old gambit and danger—*I* could not mobilize a legal defence against *her* financial resources and well she knows it. Well, no one asked me to be a psycho-analyst! . . .

July 19

. . . I have just parted from the egregious Z. It is hard to imagine anyone who qualifies better as an embodiment of verbal diarrhoea.

I am glad you were able to get the *Ulysses on the Liffey*.[1] I want to bring your Chinese Script[2] for the vacation. It is *very* good and I found it evocative even though, or because?, not always clear.

I don't know what the programme at the Hollywood Bowl is to-night. Last Saturday was Gilbert and Sullivan. Good I gather, but it must have been very depressing as there were only about 8000 there—which in the Bowl must have felt like performing in the presence of the cleaners! Rather like what I feel I am performing here . . .

July 21

. . . It is exciting to feel I shall see you soon. I had forgotten it was such ages last time but now of course it comes back to me—now it is nearly over! I am filled with astonishment and amazement at the detail with which you have gone into everything here.

July 22

Over South Dakota. Having made such an ass of myself I can hardly bear to mention it in case you want a divorce! Janet drove me to the airport and I went along to Gate 35. All went well, perfect, till I came to the last item—identity card? Rummage—no identity!—then horror dawned. I had decided to off-load junk like charge cards etc. and of course had forgotten I need my identity card for going back. Time 3.20. Plane, yes, to time. I rushed. Left my luggage with the desk and ran. Talk about the Ride to Ghent! Taxi—Homewood and back! I couldn't do the Sherlock Holmes as they have no sovereigns, and while "Dollar if you do it!" doesn't sound bad, it does not sound as good as "Cabby! A golden sovereign!" Well, on the whole I did not lose my head too—would that have been worse or better?—so I thought I might as well pick up Julian's Bible now I was weighed

[1] Richard Ellmann, Faber & Faber Ltd., 1972.
[2] *Chinese Characters*, J. Weiger, Dover Publications, Inc., N.Y.

in. Fortunately I knew exactly where I had put the cards. We were back with five minutes to spare—the last passenger after leftover seats were taken up. It is wonderful what it is to take a load off your mind, but I can't advocate putting it *on* for the pleasure of taking it off again.

It is a terribly bumpy flight. I always hope they have nailed the wings on properly. Two people on board, it has just been announced, were married an hour before boarding. Congrats—a bit half-hearted I thought.

Midnight, Pacific Time. I feel as if I have had a good night's rest—it must be because I go to sleep so suddenly, violently and completely. The film has been antique Chaplin, but I could not be bothered with it although, like all he does, he is a natural clown. He, Buster Keaton and Harold Lloyd were the only real, natural clowns, although in their time there was a cult of blowing them up to a great deal more. Still, a clown *is* somebody—Grock, Herb Williams come to mind. Grock I have heard was not so good in his native language—I never saw him except in England where on the stage he was silent and very funny. Sometimes I think my real trouble is having very easily a reputation which I don't and cannot possibly deserve, even in my wildest dreams. Do Presidents of the U.S., prime ministers and such feel that? Or perhaps they feel they earn their keep because they are liable to be bumped off—'risk pay' in other words. The L.A. Times is making a fuss of the Trades Unions' alleged threat to strike against the Law Court decisions. If it is true it ought to be made a fuss of—either the judges or the union leaders need removal. The government and its instruments must govern or they are not doing their job; and then who is to do it? It won't be long now—about another hour and a half. The sun is fully up. My goodness, it's time I saw you. It really seems to have been an age. Well—how are you?[1]

[1] This was the last letter he wrote to me; we were not separated again during the remaining seven years of his life.

THE OTHER SIDE OF GENIUS

II

Letters
To
Parthenope, Julian and Nicola

This bird 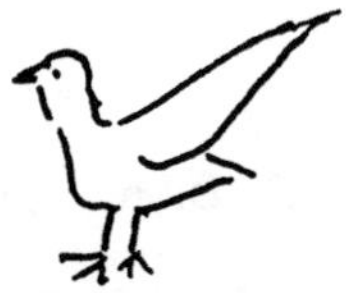 flew with us from ENGLAND to France 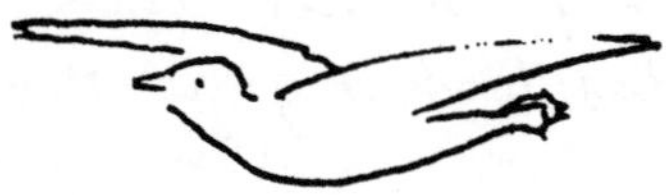 like this. Sometimes it had a rest like this → 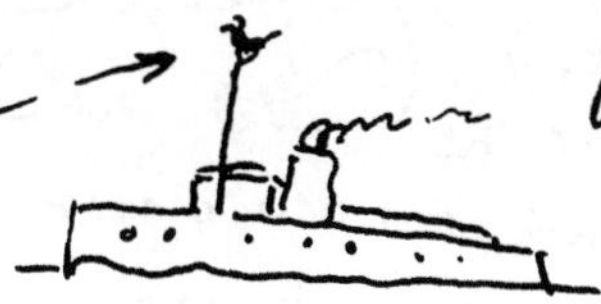 by standing on the mast of the ship. When it got to France it tidied itself up 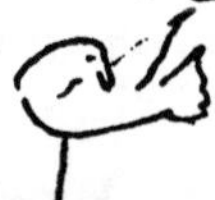 by standing on one leg and tickling itself under its wing with its beak. Then it flew back to 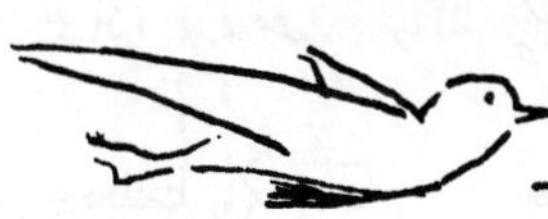 England again. Bye bye from Daddy.

1959

I thought I would send you a drawing of a rabbit 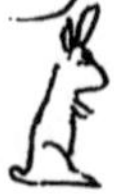 who is sitting up to see if he can find his old friend Henry. Henry's real name is Mister Edward Bear but Bunny, which is what Henry calls the rabbit, always calls Henry, Henry. Here is Henry lying on his back on a lawn covered 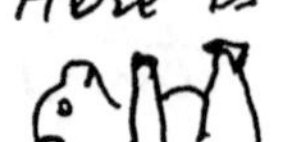 with daisies looking at the blue sky because he says it reminds him of Bunny's blue eyes. He is very fond of Bunny as you can see. He is giving Bunny a daisy he picked for her. Behind Bunny is the sea with a sailing boat which I could not draw very well because I could not see it properly. I think it must be near where Julian used to swim because I think those are the old Harry rocks where the arrow is pointing. Henry says he will take Bunny in the train.

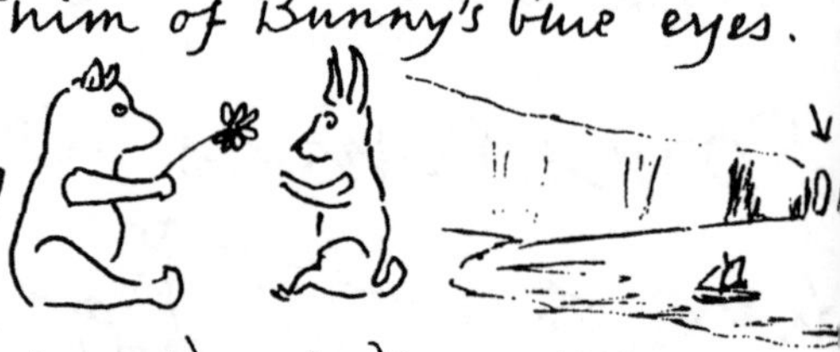

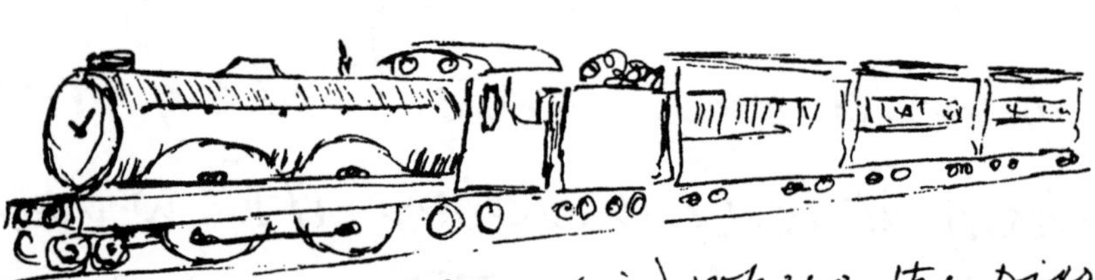

and then if they can find where the pier is they will go to see the man to go on his boat.

Goodbye till I see you later darling with love from Daddy.

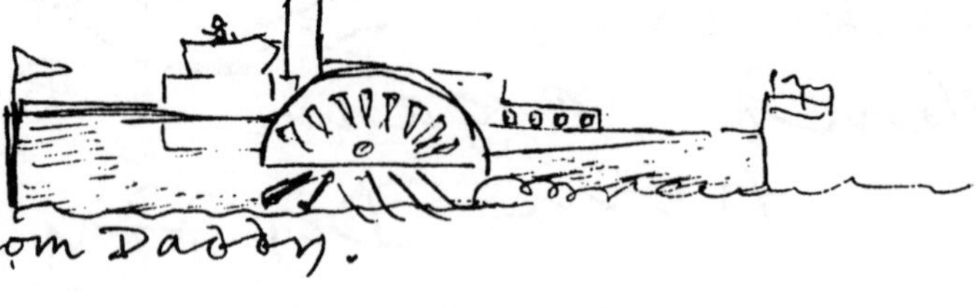

* * *

It was lovely to have the oranges from you. I like oranges very much but they are nicer because you were so kind to send them. When they dust the room here they turn a handle on the bed and this makes wheels come down so they can push the bed with me in it and I have a fine ride to the other side of the room. They call the rooms here wards. Then a very nice fat lady comes and pushes a big thing that looks like an enormous iron cake. This whirls round and polishes the floor making a lovely noise as if you were being chased by a motor bus. You can see the lady likes doing it very much indeed. And it stops sick people thinking about their illness because they are thinking what that lovely noise can be.

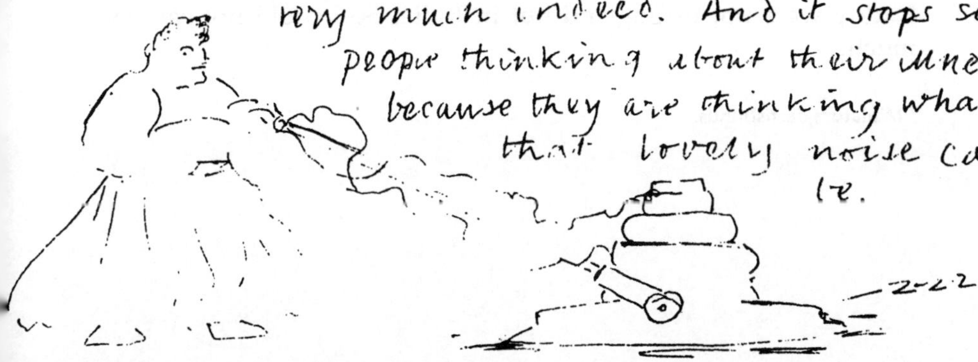

Goodbye my dear I hope I shall come back and see you all soon. With love from Daddy.

1962

In my room in Harley Street there is a small window. I keep it open so as to have plenty of fresh air. But now a pigeon has built its nest just above where it opens. And the pigeon has some eggs and is hatching out a brood of young ones. I don't know how the mother bird is going to find food for them when they come. I hope they will not make too much noise. My patients won't like it if they do.

We are all looking forward to the holidays except Mummy. Mummy does not look forward to them because she has no holidays to look forward to. In fact when our holidays come she works harder then ever. Queer, isn't it? I'm glad I'm not a mummy.

Linnet[1] looks thin and eats a lot. Dimple[1] looks fat but Linnet eats twice as much as Dimple. They both seem very well, and are looking forward to barking a lot. I suppose it's their idea of a holiday.

* * *

I wonder if there are others in your form who saw the Circus, or Jimmy Edwards in *Cinderella,* or *The Mikado?* I remember how the others at school used to talk about the theatres they had been to, but when I was small I was not often taken because my Mummy and Daddy were not in England but in India. So I could not say very much.

[1] Miniature dachshunds.

1963

We have a family of starlings who decided to live under the balcony outside the lounge. This week-end the first of the young ones left the nest; it was very interesting to see what happened. The young starling went on the rose bed. Then the mother bird came with some food. But instead of giving it to him she held it in her beak and made the baby chase her on to the lawn. Then she jumped into the air and fluttered her wings as if to say, "Look! This is how you do it!" He then took off after her and flew, low down, to the yew hedge. I suppose she gave him the food then as a prize, but we did not see that. And so it went on. He had to work hard for each bit. It was like little Tommy Tucker but this time he had to fly not sing, and it was for his breakfast, not his supper.

Then the mother took something more to the nest but she would not give it them for all their squawking and hullabuloo. It looked as if she were trying to make one get hold of the bit in her beak and then pull him out. But the babies would not take it like that. In the end she coaxed another one out. And then the lesson started all over again.

Last night Mummy and I went to a party in an old house in Hampstead.[1] First we met the other guests and saw some of the beautiful things in the house. There were harpsichords, guitars, an Indian stringed instrument that looked as if a vegetable marrow had been made into a boat, some virginals, one of the earliest grand pianos, and two spinets. They were all *old* musical instruments. You were allowed to touch all of them except a harpsichord that used to belong to the great composer Handel who wrote the *Messiah* which you will hear one day; it is a very magnificent piece of music called an Oratorio. After half an hour we went into one of the big rooms to hear a concert. There was one of the best harpsichord players in England[2] and he accompanied a soprano singer. She was very big and had a big voice and sang a lot of songs written by John Dowland and other famous song writers of Shakespeare's time. Her voice was rather like our dishwasher when it has gone wrong and you could hardly hear the harpsichord because she sang so loud, but otherwise it was very nice. Then the man played the harpsichord alone and that was beautiful: it looked very difficult.

Then a lady who goes around to different countries to learn about their music, played a lute which is a stringed instrument with

[1] Fenton House.
[2] Ralph Kirkpatrick.

fourteen strings and looks like a huge melon, and sang songs from the Outer Hebrides. She played a drum which had been given her in Mexico and sang a song to their god of Thunder and Rain. She was very clever with the drum which looked like a big waste-paper basket, and made high notes and low notes. It sounded like a thunderstorm with big drops of rain falling. Then we had supper: chicken and salmon mousse (salmon pounded into a slush) and Russian salad and strawberries and ice cream. Then Mummy and I came home.

* * *

I hope you are working hard and playing hard and sleeping soft and laughing hard at other people's jokes—you aren't supposed to laugh at your own because it looks conceited. But you can laugh up your sleeve although I have never seen anyone do it. The villains or the heroes of stories do it and very soon after, or before, some one says "Ah hah!" (not ha, ha, ha, haa) but in a nasty kind of way meaning "Sucks to you!"

* * *

I hope you are enjoying your term. I always thought the summer term very nice because we used to have lots of swimming and we could go out for walks in the country when we got to the Main School. But not in the Preparatory School because, like yours, our prep school was in a town. I did not like walks then because we went with the master and if we lagged behind we had to do a lot of difficult sums as a punishment.

* * *

The barn owl has moved off. Mummy is glad but I am sorry: still he didn't seem to want any humans in his barn

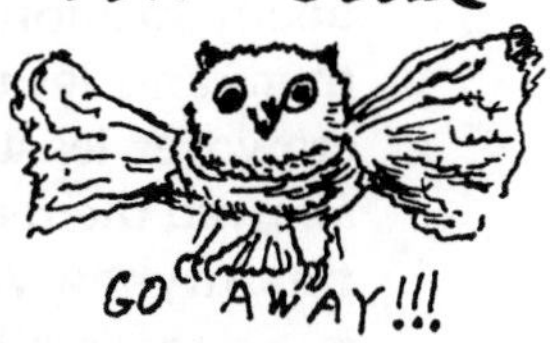

and it would be awkward for Mummy to be dive-bombed and sworn at whenever she came in and wanted to do some gardening. This is a picture of Shadow being talked to by Mumm

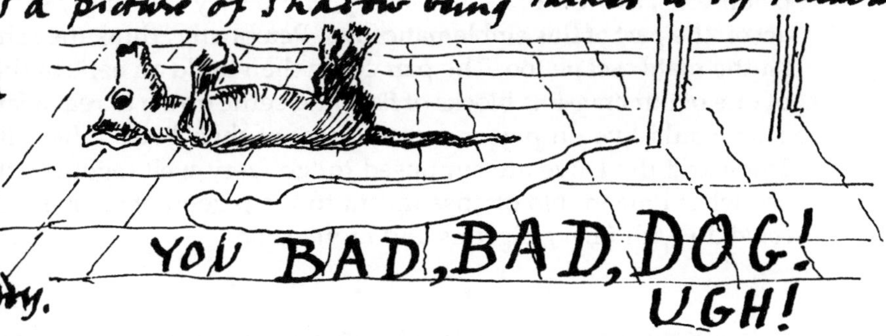

Much love from us all.
from Daddy.

* * *

All my memories of homesickness are of it as the most ghastly feeling I ever knew—a sort of horrible sense of impending disaster without any idea what it was or even any words in which to express it. Not much better is what I think of as the 2 a.m. feeling when some horrible worry comes on you with such force that it makes your blood run cold. One might write an anthology but it would require skill, almost amounting to genius, to begin to recall the absolute dread that comes on these occasions. But I believe it is from one's ability to stand having such feelings and ideas that mental growth eventually comes.

Today was another fine day and we went into the park in the morning. There we saw a vast concourse, guessed it was *the* Eagle,[1] and joined in. He was in a tree surveying us all and no doubt thinking

[1] It had escaped from Regent's Park Zoo.

we would all be far better on the other side of some bars. On the ground was his mate, tethered, a dead rabbit and a contraption of nets. After he had watched the pantomime for a while he lost interest and flew off. We all crowded in and trod on the nets and gaped in a booby fashion when the keepers tried to persuade us to move off them and let them take the gear away. As I imagine that half the crowd at least don't want him to be caught I don't think anyone allowed themselves to be incommoded unduly by the keeper's chagrin. Anyhow you can hardly blame an eagle if it is tepid about landing in a very small trap set in the middle of a crowd of 2000 people just for the sake of some dead rabbit and the uncertain welcome of his very eagle-eyed, handsome, and well taloned wife. Earlier he had carefully killed and eaten a muscovy duck on the lawns of the American Embassy; which, when you think the duck was almost certainly communist in view of its nationality, was a very sportingly symbolic act on the part of this emblematic fowl. Personally I think they should let the mate escape too. The pair could then build an eerie at the top of one of our crag-like blocks of flats and settle down to rear a family. They could live on pigeons for the rest of their lives. After all, the Eagle and the Dove are supposed to 'go' very well together, if you see what I mean. No offense meant to the pigeon of course, but we *could* do with fewer pigeons and more eagles.

*   *   *

It is terrible to skim over a job and get a superficial smattering that is nothing more than a facile covering up for ignorance. It is an easy but awful habit to get into because you then go on bluffing even if there is no need to do so. Don't make the mistake of thinking any worthwhile job that is done properly will ever feel easy. Unfortunately, fooling one's self and others is both easy and *not* worthwhile.

*   *   *

I know what you mean when you speak of feeling at home with the 'scruffy' people. Unfortunately there *are* people with scruffy *minds* and they do not obligingly declare that fact by wearing distinctive clothes. But I think you should be able to penetrate the disguises if you remember that disguises exist. It's like obscurity in literature: genuine people are obscure only because they cannot make it clearer; others want you to think they must be clever if they are incomprehensible.

*   *   *

I have been getting up my paper which I give to the Society on Wednesday next.[1] Although I know pretty well what I want to say, it has meant time to send out the typed and duplicated copy and more time producing the version I want to speak. I never read what I have written or print what I have said if I can possibly avoid it. They are two such very different things that I think it most important to treat them differently. If you are speaking you must be repetitive which is quite wrong for the written communication.

It is an old tradition that the British are phlegmatic. The Elizabethans were certainly a more cheerful lot though they had plenty to worry about. But they hadn't an Empire and I don't think this country has ever taken kindly to having one. but it is different, if you have never had one, from feeling you have had one and lost it. When we settle down we may concentrate quite cheerfully on minding our own business—it could certainly do with a bit of minding anyway.

I have almost finished all the writing I want to do for my book.[2] But the last chapter is important and therefore tricky. And then comes all the correction and excision which I find a bit tiresome. I never realized before I tried that you don't just write a book—you have to *make* it as well.

* * *

Mummy and I are both feeling a bit limp recovering from the Jubilee dinner at the Savoy—or rather from the efforts required. Mummy had a terrific job as Chairman of the Ladies Committee responsible for the arrangements—the seating and proper precedence was a headache in itself, and that was only a part of it. We had to get there about half an hour before just to see all was in order and that we had not got the wrong night or something equally horrifying. The dining room with its flowers looked very good—a long top table and then lots of round tables holding ten each. Then we went upstairs to the reception room ready for the guests. At 8 p.m. they started arriving, with the Toastmaster resplendent in his red coat bawling their names as they came. We spent the next half hour shaking hands—three hundred of them. My smile began to become a bit sickly fairly early in the proceedings. Then we trooped down to dinner, Mummy and I leading. The Toastmaster was a bit shocked as I said there would be no grace, whether because he relied

[1] 'The Grid'. Published in *Two Papers*, Imago Editora, Rio de Janeiro, 1977.
[2] *Transformations*, Heinemann Medical Books, 1965.

on grace as a signal to start serving the meal or because of religious scruples I don't know. We had turtle soup; truite meunière; tournedos; and a sweet which was an ice-cream covered in egg-white froth baked in an oven and served with cherries in burning kirsch. Of course the ice-cream, being insulated by the egg white, was frozen stiff and the rest of it hot. It was a good dinner only spoiled for me by my having to be the Big Noise. Then the Toastmaster in thunderous tones announced, "Ladies and Gentlemen: pray silence for your President." (Come to think of it—I am a sort of Psychoanalytic Pope!) and I gave the toast of 'The Queen'. A couple of minutes later I was up again and made my speech. We then had a speech from Dr Sylvia Payne on the history of the previous fifty years of the Society, and another from James Strachey. Then a speech by the representative of the International Psycho-Analytical Association, and after that telegrams from various parts of the world wishing us well. At about 11.10 we broke up to get to the car. Mummy and I finally got home to bed by about 2 a.m. Hence the lassitude.

1964

Be careful not to mistake plants having their winter rest for weeds or dead. They will soon look very much alive when the sap begins to flow and they wake from their winter sleep. One day in your Latin you may read Virgil's IVth Georgic where he tells about an old man who used to grow a few lilies and verbena and always had the best vegetables and fruit earlier than anyone else.

* * *

Nicola stayed away from school on Friday as she felt sick but felt perfectly well all day so I think she must have had a bad attack of school-sickness—you know, longing to get back to school ha! ha! and ever so keen on her hoam werk.

* * *

Last night Mummy and I went to see *Lawrence of Arabia*. With one ten minute interval it lasted from 7.15 to 10.50 so it was quite a piece. The desert photography was magnificent in every way: beautiful colour and superbly done. So I suppose was the story, if it is admitted that it has to be interpreted by photographs of actors acting. But when the drama lies in character, this is not good enough and no one has yet produced, in U.S. or Britain, film that goes below the surface. With Allenby, the greatest man of them all, Feisal, Lawrence, Auda, you need the Rodin technique as opposed to Praxiteles. Still, we both enjoyed it for the sheer magnificence of the desert, and the human beings did not spoil it. But that is not fair—the acting *was* good. But it is difficult for an actor to act a shy man who acts always as if he were acting a part as an extremely 'ham' hero. It's too complicated. And of course Allenby, who really *was* great, came out as nobody at all—the mess-waiter acting the part of a general in the Officers Mess Christmas rag. It was however very well worth seeing.

* * *

We have been watching Dr Who: awful tosh of course, but made so much worse by the characters all being quite uiniformly unsympathetic. Various robots appear but the machines are at least metallic whereas the flesh and blood is wooden.

Julian said the other day, "What a happy place school would be if masters did not think they had to bash the lessons into you." I thought it was a very acute observation but unhappily school masters do not make it themselves. So many people go to school longing to learn and end up hating it. But of course there is always someone bashing the masters to bash.

How difficult it is to realize that with certain books one does not 'read' them—one has to have an emotional experience of reading them. This seems so slow compared with the easy slick reading, especially if you feel you have exams to pass, that it is very difficult to give one's self the time and other conditions necessary for it—especially the time.

* * *

Most nations at least pretend to worship their illustrious dead although—

'De tous ces défunts cockolores
Le moral Fenelon,
Michel Ange et Johnson (Le Docteur),
Sont les plus awful bores.'

But I agree that the French, and the Italians even more, do seem able to live or think it worth trying. Of the Germans the French say that they know how to die, but *not* how to live.

* * *

The Pirandello which we saw on Friday is *Six Characters in Search of an Author*. It is a very good play, but what was so interesting to me was the clarity with which Pirandello brought out the author's dilemma, namely the struggle of the ideas to find expression and then the problem of making them true without their being so unaesthetically expressed that they are incomprehensible or too unacceptable on the one hand, or, on the other 'artistic' or acceptable but so distorted as to lack all honesty or integrity. The ending is too melodramatic I have always thought, but even that was well done. It could be argued that a good play will always get through but I think it indisputable that the better the play the more there is to get lost on the way.

* * *

There is only one thing that matters to us and has ever mattered to me, and that is that you should have in yourself a knowledge of yourself and others that will make you able to make the best of what life holds for you. To do this I have always realized you need to experiment and learn for yourself. I know that life can be very hard and can stifle growth; all I want is that it should not be needlessly so. Present happiness owes much to previous drudgery, and future happiness may depend on present drudgery. There is no virtue in drudgery, but if you can face it with equanimity, *if you must*, then it is an invaluable stand-by and no amount of ability or luck can make up for it.

Imagination is very valuable. Without it you cannot see your way, but it must not become a *substitute* for real life. One *can* be so crippled by the mere grind of finding bread and butter, and the pain of competition for the mere necessities of life, that it is impossible for one's talent to find itself. It is equally true that you can be stifled by over-ease. There is no question of my being upset by any choice you make except one—a choice that led you to retreat into imagining a good life instead of finding your own way to it. Milton says, 'Taught by the heavenly muse to venture down the dark descent, and up to reascend though hard and rare' when talking of his journey—and that was tough enough in all conscience, but made tougher by his knowledge of his own greatness and the burden that put on him. But this is true even of ordinariness, if one can call a knowledge so extra-ordinary as knowledge of one's ordinariness, 'ordinary'. One will always crave 'ordinary' sun and air and rain and cloud and food and happiness. If imagination helps you to find it, it is a fine thing. But it is a curse if a belief in some 'extra-ordinary' life puts a barrier between you and it. Believe me, I should hate it more than I can say if I felt that anything I said or did led you to find some 'success' that stood between you and these great and simple things. If you read very carefully the opening of Book III of *Paradise Lost*, you will realize that Milton was not talking about his blindness only, though most people (even the ones who ought to know better) think so, but about the inner light; that is *his* way of putting it. He uses the language of his time and beliefs to express himself, but *what* he expresses is knowledge that only a great man has and which transcends the accidents of his time and circumstances. As you grow older your experience will teach you more and more of the great depth of his understanding. Only one who knows could say what he says about love (in Book IV, 'Here love his golden shafts emploies—'). I do *not* wish anything for you but that you should find yourself and *your* life.

* * *

Depression and failure are a part of every life even the most happy and successful—I might say *especially* of the most happy and successful; it is the price you pay for joy and success if they come your way. But the price you pay for trying to *evade* failure and depression is ten times worse. To start off with, happiness and success are very good things—*in their own right*. It is quite another matter if you are compelled to be 'happy' and 'successful' because you fear failure and depression. It spoils the success because you feel there is something it is hiding, and failure and depression become such bogeys that you cannot believe they are what quite ordinary people take in their stride any day of their lives. I want you to form your own judgments and make your own decisions. But I do want you to learn how to make them for the *right reasons*. All this is easy for me to write but I know of no one for whom it is easy to practise.

* * *

The other day when I was going to work I crossed Green Park and a blackbird came hopping along the path to meet me. It came right up to me; I think it must have been so tame because it was starving and hoped I had some crumbs, but I hadn't any to give the poor thing. I am glad all the snow has gone for the sake of the birds. Now it is warmer they have started fighting for territory. That means that they try to get a part of the garden for themselves so they can find plenty of food near their nests. A beautiful woodpecker was on the lawn today and he looked very fine in his new feathers and bright red cap.

* * *

When I drew the curtains just now I saw Venus and the sickle moon. Venus is the very bright star—a planet really—that shows up clearly just after the sun has set. You can see the dark part of the moon tonight because it must be lit up by light from the earth just as we can see on a night when we are brightly lit up by moonlight. It seems funny to think of earthlight instead of moonlight, doesn't it?

* * *

There was a fine green and red woodpecker on the lawn this morning. He was having no end of a time with a worm (I think)—anyway he seemed to be struggling with something big. Usually of course they tap trees for the insects in the bark. And he would hardly have had all that trouble with an ant.

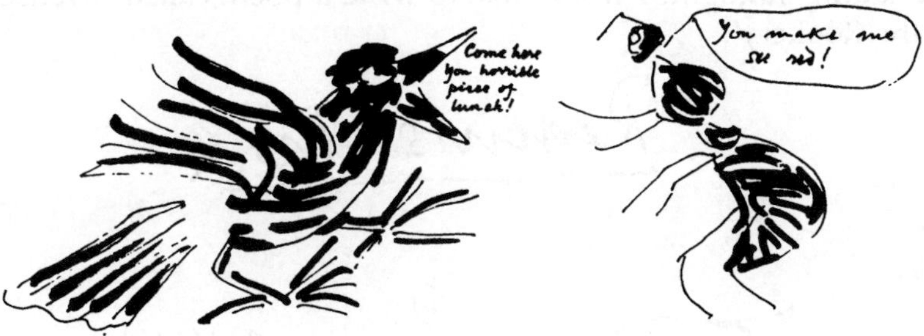
Come here you horrible piece of lunch!
You make me see red!

* * *

This morning I went to the Design Centre where they had a lot of chairs. One was a huge thing about up to my elbows like a round puff-ball. I sat on it and it sank in so that it made a lovely armchair. It was like being eaten up and swallowed by a Yorkshire pudding!

* * *

Linnet and Dimple seem to have found a big garbage supply and both are looking stout. One of them brought in a huge bone and left it on the carpet for Mummy as a present. Mummy didn't seem to want it. It would have been awkward if she had cooked it for our lunch.

Mummy is very busy indeed running the house as usual *and* doing all the work about the new one, measuring carpets and rooms and places where things have to go. I don't know how she manages. And just now she is correcting my next book.[1]

[1] *Transformations, see also* f.n. p.175.

1965

After we had been to see the armour and some paintings at Hertford House (the Wallace Collection where you drew some of the daggers one day) we walked back through the park. Another dog chased a crow yesterday. This time the rook made a terrible squawking and seemed most upset about it. It's a pity they don't seem to be tame at all, not even to want to feed. They are so respectable in their glossy black Sunday clothes. I love it when they sit high up in their rookeries in the evening and caw their good-nights to each other in the fading sunlight. I would like to write a poem called 'Evensong at the Rookery'.

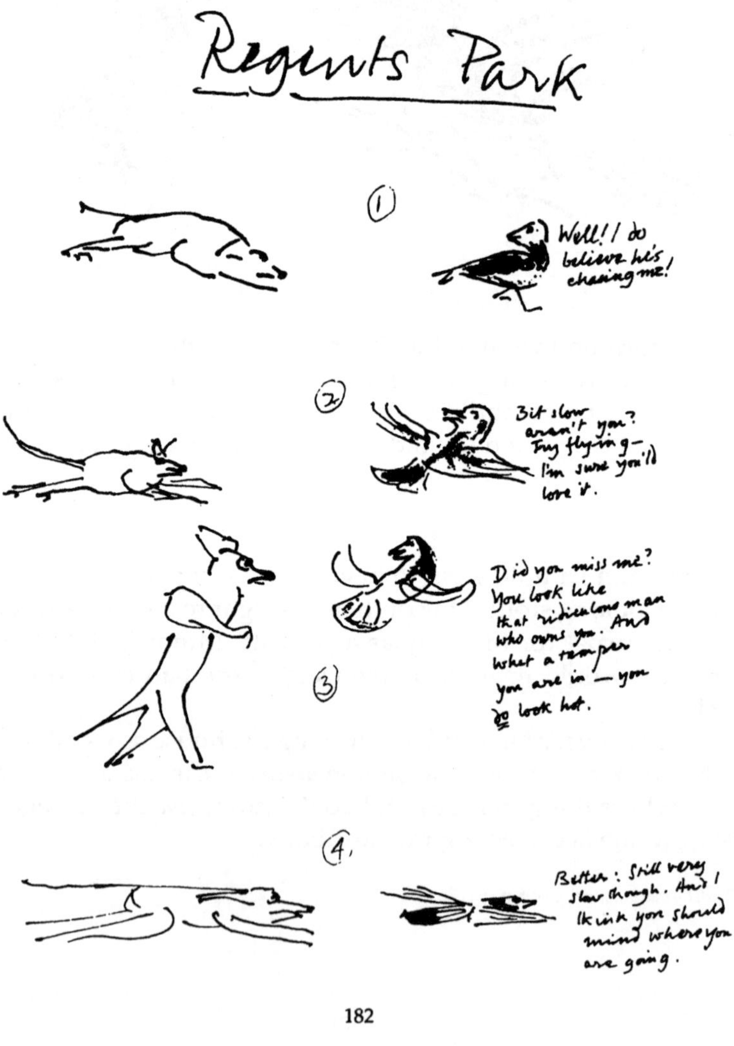

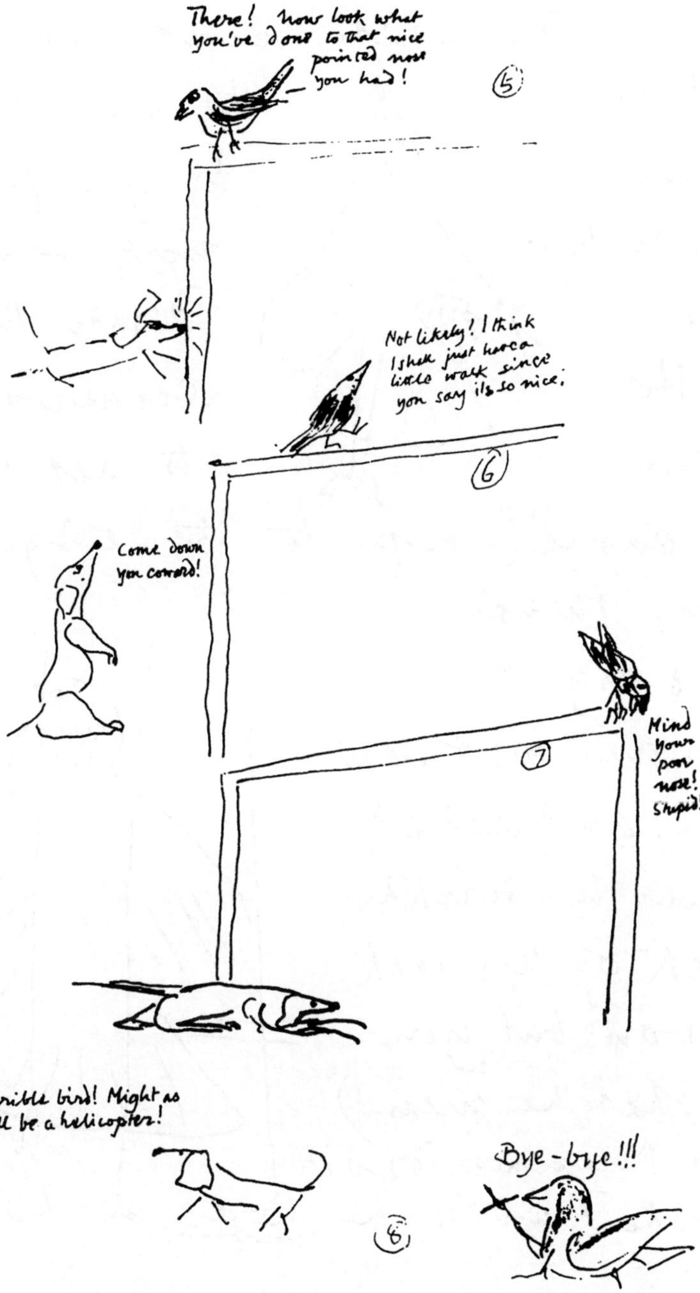
There! now look what you've done to that nice pointed nose you had!
5
Not likely! I think I shall just have a little walk since you say it's so nice.
6
Come down you coward!
Mind your poor nose! Stupid!
7
Horrible bird! Might as well be a helicopter!
Bye-bye!!!
8

* * *

...The white cockatoo was still there — the one that danced to you (a bit like this but not very as I can't draw him very well. He seemed lonely and glad to see mummy

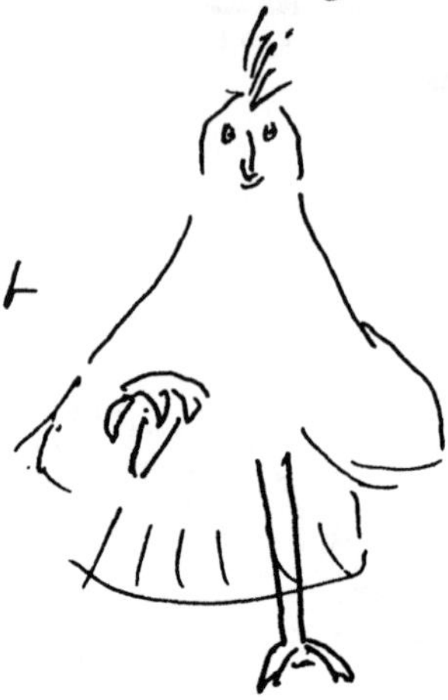

So he came up to the edge of the cage, turned his head right round and looked at heaven, and asked mummy to scratch the back of his neck. (Not in words but you know what he meant) When Mummy did it he looked as if he *was* in heaven!

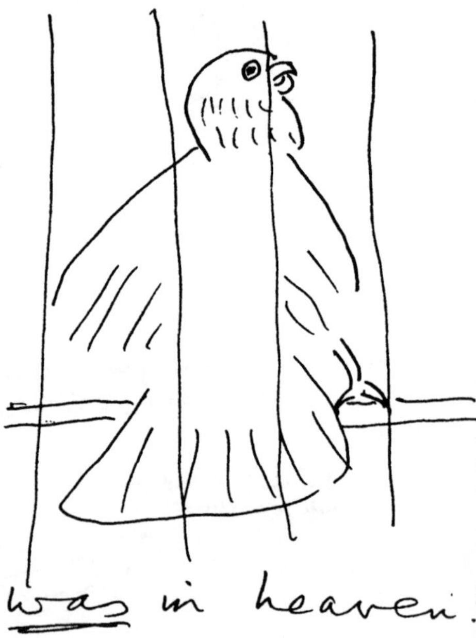

As you can see I can't draw Kangaroos or fawns but I wanted to because when I was going in to the Park by the path that runs along the enclosure for the red-rumped Ajouti. (only one is certainly black rumped) I saw the Kangaroo kneeling down and the fawn (which looks like the Devil in my sketch) was standing over it and licking its face and ears in a most loving and tender way. They looked very pretty and I wished you could have seen them. I have never seen such a thing before though I have heard of a big mastiff bitch bringing up some tiger-cubs as her babies till they become too rough. "Oh mummy I love you _so_ much I could eat.... oh heavens! Where's mummy gone?" you can imagine them saying "No THANK you (UGH!) I'm off!" says mummy bitch.

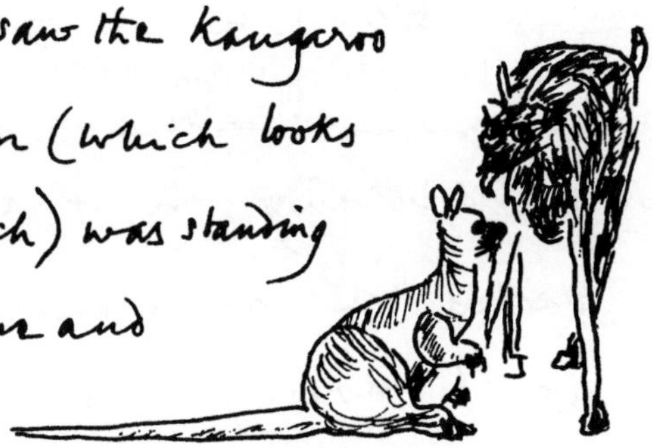

*   *   *

As I am sitting here in the lounge writing I can see the garden trellis with

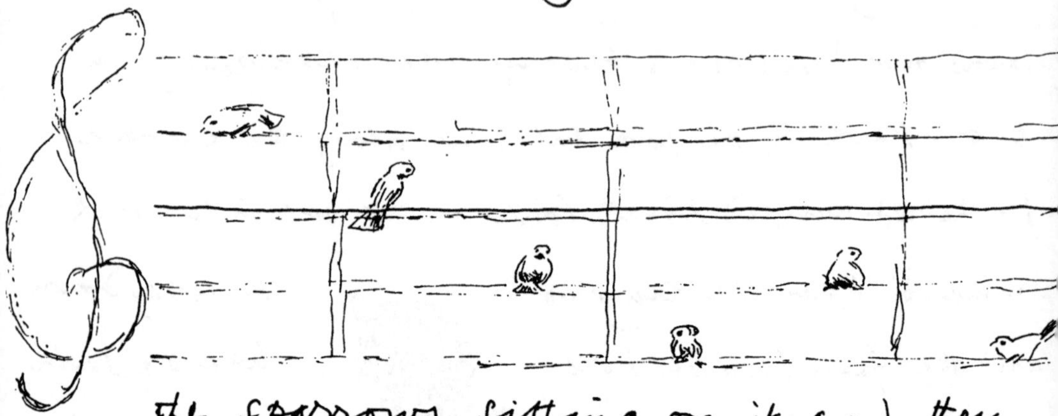

the sparrows sitting on it and they look just like notes on a musical stave. But I don't think I have got the curley-cue right. It would be rather fun to "play" the sparrows on the trellis on the piano. Perhaps they would form themselves into a musical composition as one flew off and another came.

Last night Mummy and I went to a big dinner at the Connaught Rooms.[1] Mummy had been working very hard arranging where

[1] To celebrate the completion of the publication of the Standard Edition of Freud's works, translated by James Strachey.

everyone had to sit. As there were 380 people to dinner it was Quite a job to arrange it so that the one's who hated each other did not come together and the fat ones and the thin ones came together. (Otherwise two fat ones would not have enough room and two thin ones would be leaving a space). Then the greedy ones needed to be next to the ones who could not stand the food (ugh!) so that they could have extra and nothing would be wasted. There was a Toast Master. He wore a gorgeous scarlet uniform and had an enormous VOICE. You might think his job would be to bawl out "LOOK OUT! the toast's BURNING!" but it isn't. He just stands at the door when you come in and goes "Dr AND Mrs BION!!!". Mummy and I got in first so he couldn't do it to us. Anyhow he gave up after about 20 people so I think he can't have fancied having to shout 360 more names.

Mummy sat between Sir Frank Francis who is librarian to the British Museum which is the greatest library in the World and Sir Frederick Hoare who was LORD MAYOR of LONDON — like Dick Whittington but he hadn't got a cat with him and he didn't bring his dinner tied up in a red bandana handkerchief carried at the end of his stick which he rested on his shoulder. That is how I always see LORDS Mayor of London. I sat between Lady Hoare and Mrs Strachey. Mrs Strachey didn't eat anything but

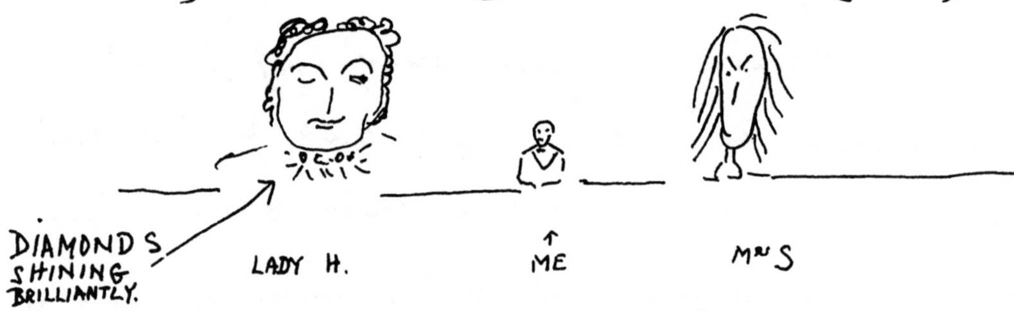

she is extremely intelligent and only has one or two good ideas for dinner. She is very nice and only looks a bit sad because she had to bring her own good ideas. Lady Hoare as you can see is very intelligent AND brilliant. After dinner we all talked and wandered around and Mummy and I left to get home by midnight. Mummy wore a shiny blue dress with a large trailing thing at the back and long white elbow length gloves and gold and white lace shoes. She looked very smart indeed. I wore a dinner jacket. I also had to give a book to Mr Strachey and Miss Frend which I did without dropping them, tripping up over the microphone, falling flat on my face, bursting into tears, or shouting with laughter because all their faces look so funny like plaice on a fish-mongers slab. All of which I am . . .

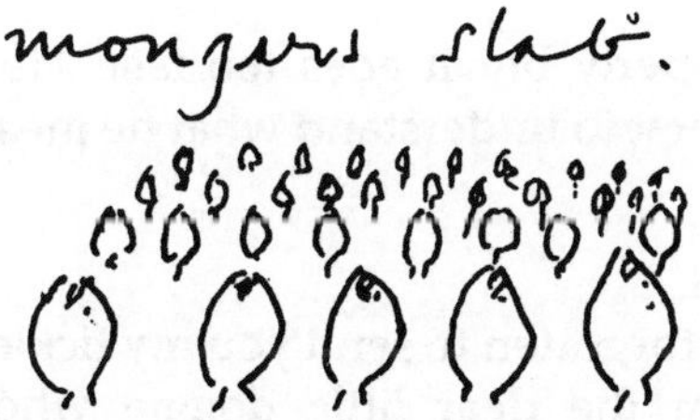

afraid I shall do before I actually come to the dinner or whatever it at which I am supposed to speak.

* * *

Bad writing is as bad as mumbling instead of talking because it looks as if you expected others to read what you can't be bothered to write. Or listen to what you can't be bothered to say.

There are still baby ducks, geese and coots in the Park. I've tried

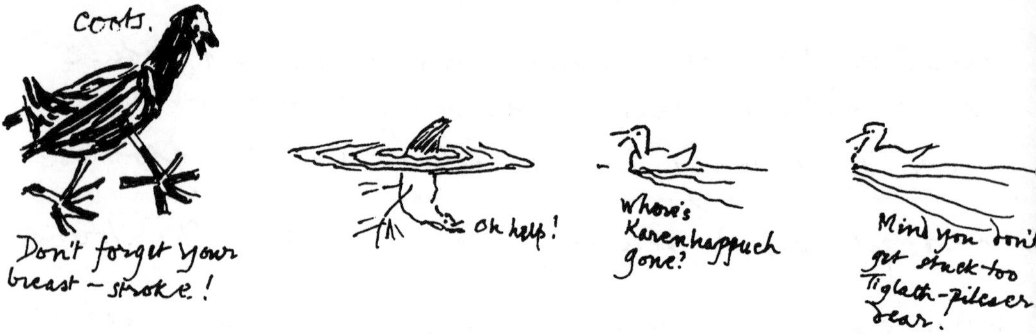
Coots.
Don't forget your breast-stroke!
Oh help!
Where's Karenhappuch gone?
Mind you don't get stuck too Tiglath-pileser dear.

to draw some coots.[1] Of course I am not sure but I think coots do have long names because their family name—coot—is so terribly short and it must be very disappointing to have a short name like 'coot'. Before you know anyone has spoken to you it's all over so to speak.

Last night Mummy and I went to see Perry, or Perry thought so and was glad to see us and about fifty other people who had come to see him. He received the guests from under the table and then went round and spoke to each one separately. Ticklee-tum, ticklee-tum he said as he graciously rolled over on to his back. I am sorry I

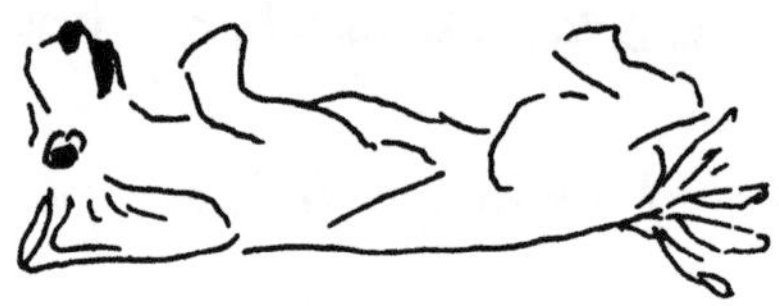

cannot show his tail wagging properly but it goes too fast. He is smiling because Mummy was the first to understand what he meant by Ticklee-tum.

P.S.

I don't know why your Daddy has forgotten to send you my ticklee-tums too. You remember?—I am the dear little doggie whom everyone thinks so SWEET—which I was and still am. I allow the Sandlers to look after me. In Circus Road. And you promised to take me for a walk. I am a Jack Russell Terrier. THE Jack Russell Terrier. Hoping your Headmistress Tickles your Tum too. Just lie on your back and stick your paws in the air like I do and I'm sure she will make you top of the school.

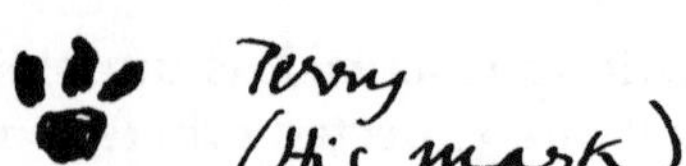

[1] Keren Happuch, Job's third and youngest daughter.
[2] Tiglath Pileser, an Assyrian king, eighth century B.C.

Mouse's fare refunded

FROM OUR CORRESPONDENT

WAKEFIELD, SEPT. 18

A 7d. fare charged for George, a four-week-old pet white mouse, for the six-mile bus journey from Wakefield to the village of Woolley, Yorkshire, was refunded yesterday. The owner of the mouse, Judith Sharp, aged 10, received a formal apology from a bus company official.

An inspector of the West Riding Automobile Company drove to the girl's home in The Crescent, Morley, near Leeds, and asked to see George.

The girl said: "He told me he was very sorry about George having to pay his fare, and gave me back the 7d."

She returned to England from Canada with her parents, Mr. and Mrs. Edward Sharp only a month ago.

CONDUCTOR INSISTED

After being given the mouse by a cousin, the girl took it on a bus. George measures 3½in. from his nose to the tip of his tail, but the conductor insisted that livestock must be paid for. He told the girl's grandfather, Mr. Donald Barker, who was with her, that unless the fare was paid they would have to get off. So Mr. Barker gave him the 7d.—only 1d. less than the girl's fare.

Mr. Peter Daykin, transport manager of West Riding Automobile Company, said their regulations included a fare scale for livestock carried in baskets, such as pigeons or cats, but did not cover the transport of a mouse.

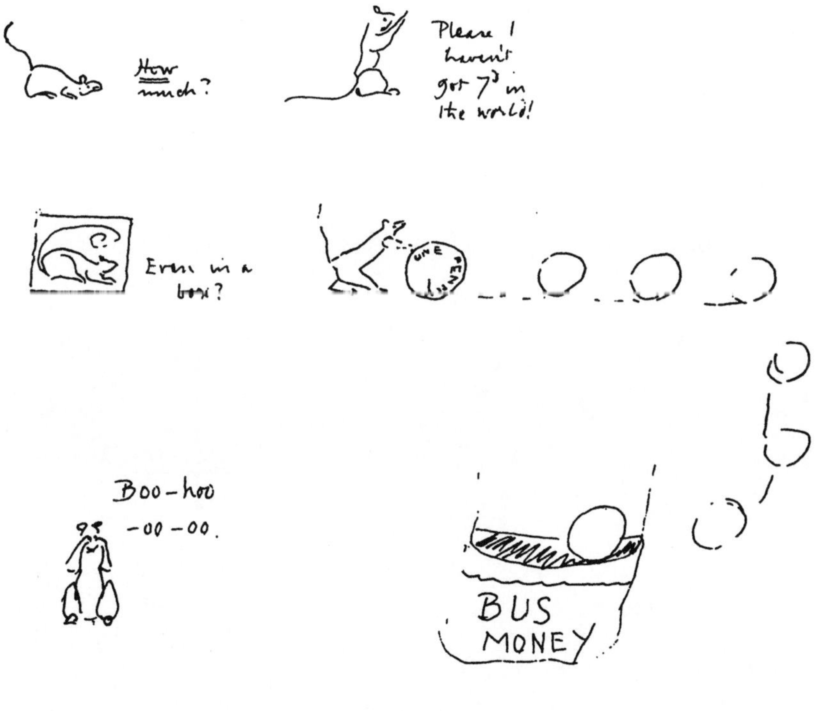
How much?
Please I haven't got 7d in the world!
Even in a box?
ONE PENNY
Boo-hoo -oo-oo.
BUS MONEY

1967

I am so sorry it is such ages since I wrote to you and that I have not replied to your very good long letters. Not counting the spelling of course, but then quite famous people like Queen Elizabeth I and Shakespeare spelled very badly. But perhaps that was reasonable when most people didn't spell at all. Elizabeth *wrote* very beautifully. The great advantage of not spelling very well was that you could spell as you felt. For example, 'i thinke hee is a fatte-hedded fule'. Much better than 'I think he is a fat-headed fool', don't you think?

* * *

I'm sending you some of my thumb prints. It makes an awful mess of your thumb. In fact it makes an awful mess. I like the one bathing best—the wet one.

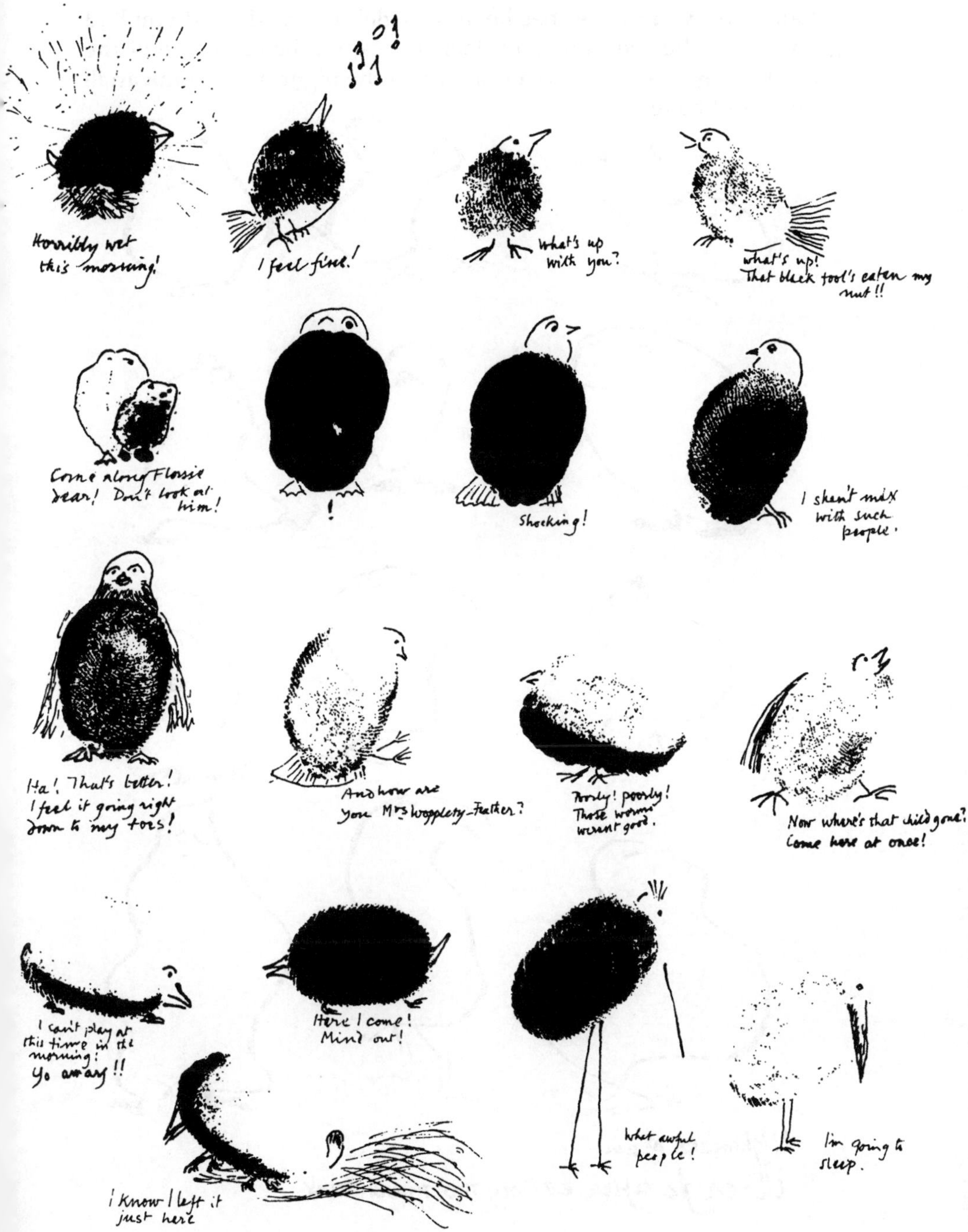
Horribly wet this morning!
I feel fine!
What's up with you?
What's up! That black tool's eaten my nut!!
Come along Flossie dear! Don't look at him!
!
Shocking!
I shan't mix with such people.
Ha! That's better! I feel it going right down to my toes!
And how are you Mrs Wopplety-Feather?
Poorly! poorly! Those worms weren't good.
Now where's that child gone? Come here at once!
I can't play at this time in the morning! Go away!!
Here I come! Mind out!
What awful people!
I'm going to sleep.
I know I left it just here

* * *

I am sorry your locker has been 'illeagle'. It sounds as if you had got the bird, but perhaps your locker escaped the eagle eye of the prefects. Anyhow I enclose a drawing of the nightmare I think an ill eagle might have.

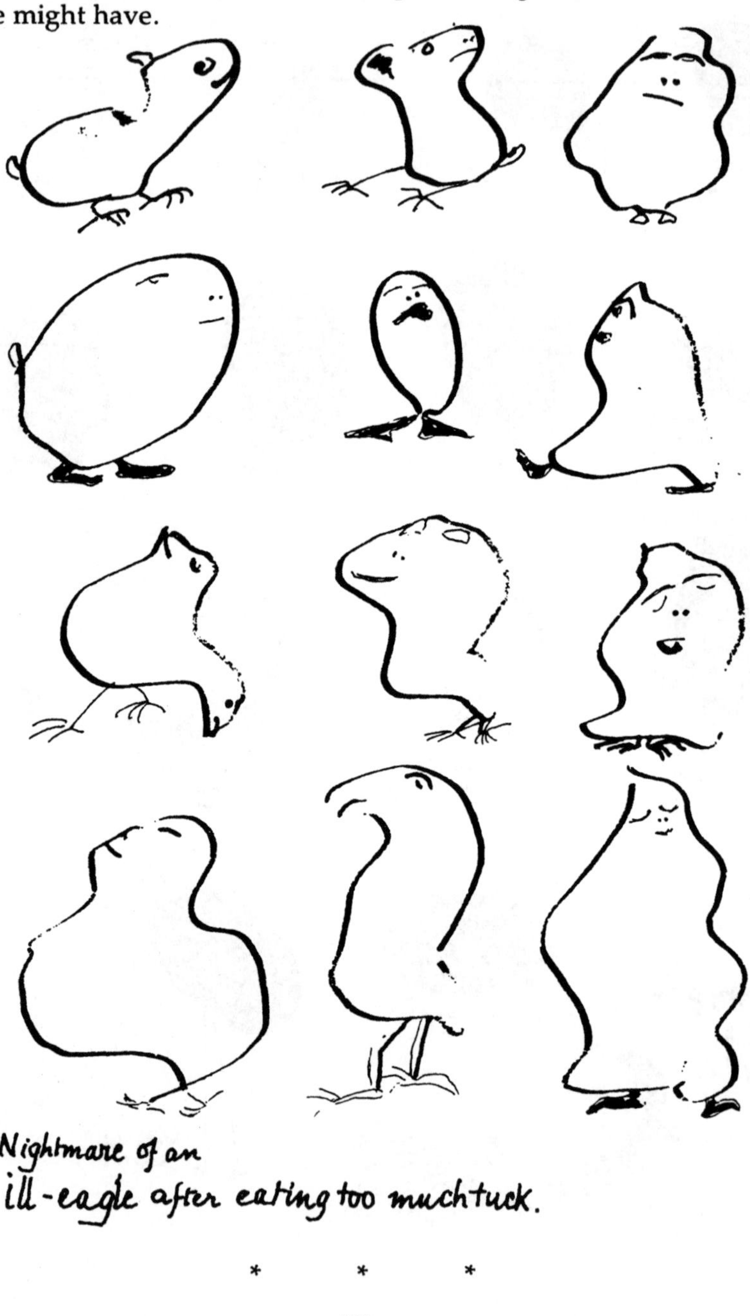

Nightmare of an
ill-eagle after eating too much tuck.

* * *

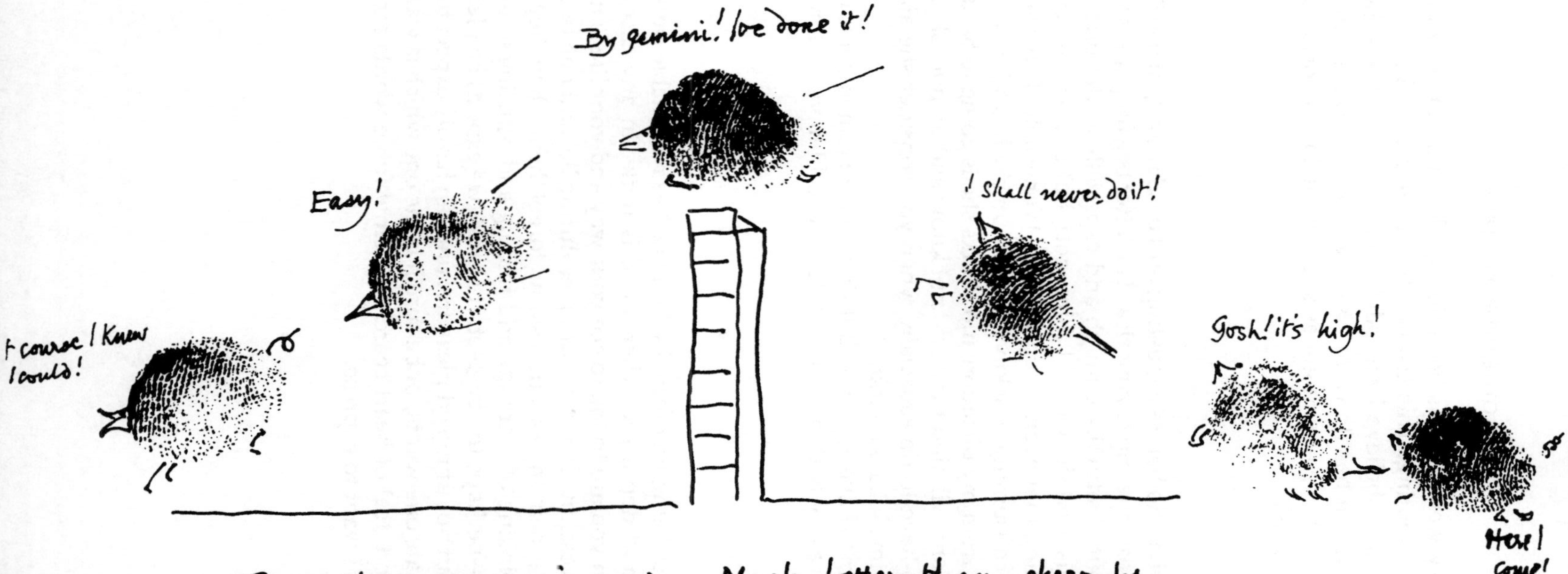
f course I knew I could!
Easy!
By gemini! Ive done it!
I shall never do it!
Gosh! it's high!
Here I come!

Thumble-wurzels jumping. Much better than sheep for counting with to go to sleep.

Kiki[1] is very well and has been doing a lot of mumble-twittering and sparrow-shouting. This last is rather rude really. She is on the balcony and has I believe been talking to a blue tit in the honeysuckle. The blue tit has flown off. Kiki was sitting up very straight, and if she was talking as straight as she sounded I am not surprised the blue tit flew off.

* * *

I have much to do before a meeting on Tuesday and, more distant but still too close, the trip to America. The latter beg for papers which are written out—naturally enough and especially at the price they want to pay (is *want* the word? I think not), but I hate it and cannot imagine sticking to it even when written. Worse still of course, it is terribly time-consuming. Luckily for me Mummy has taken it down in shorthand from my dictation and thinks she is going to be able to type it. How she will find time I do not know and do not ask. It is a terrible lot to have to do especially when you consider she already has two full-time jobs on hand.

I never seem to have any time. But since I never remember to count the ten hours a day with patients I naturally feel I haven't done any work.

* * *

It is hopeless being unaffected when one has reasonable cause for depression, and depressed when there is none. In any case, it *is* difficult when you are trying to see your way and your life is unsettled. These occasions repeat themselves during life and one tends to underestimate their unpleasantness and forget them when they have subsided. Thinking of marriage and finding and courting a mate is one of them—perhaps the biggest. It *should* (we expect) be pleasant and so it is. But not unmixed pleasure; one can hardly expect to find the kind of mate one wants, or be sure it is the one which is wanted, without a good deal of heart-searching. How futile words seem to express what I want to express.

* * *

[1] A budgerigar.

1968

Here we are in our new home. The journey was long because of head winds which made the Pan Am authorities route the plane by Mong-ray-ahl instead of the polar route. The Mong-ray-ahl-ers were very sluggish about loading petrol (gas) but perhaps this was because the temperature was 0° Fahrenheit (32 degrees of frost). I had been feeling terribly hot in my thornproof suit so walked to the rear door. All doors open but no one allowed out. Before I knew where I was I found out what 32 degrees of frost means. I thought I would not feel warm again! We had sunset for about two hours—blood-red sky. Then Los Angeles looking like a marvellous garden of flowers made out of precious stones.

On Friday it rained and on Saturday it poured—properly. No nonsense about 'rain' as in England, but the real thing as in India when I was small. Today we woke up to white frost (we *never* have frost in California) and brilliant sunshine and blue skies. I may say I bathed in the pool on Friday but it *was* cold! Bitter! I couldn't stay in, but just swam the length and back. Also a hummingbird obligingly showed up and today Mummy and I both saw it. Seems queer to have a real hummingbird mucking about in your garden; also a beautiful dove which is very tame and sits about, or walks, even if you are within a couple of yards. It doesn't like white bread but only cornflakes.

It is difficult to believe it's January. There are begonias in the garden. Green but already large strawberries, azaleas in bloom and camellias just coming out. The real pleasure though is in the blue sky and sun which we have had for the whole of the day.

* * *

Mummy and I have just had our first breakfast in the garden outside the living room. I am writing this in the same place. I don't want to make your mouth water but it is *very* nice. I had a long swim before breakfast; the pool is bright blue like the sky and the temperature during breakfast was 75° in the shade. There is a cool breeze. The blue jay came down just now to scold Grandma because he thought she was trying to pinch his strawberries. He was in fact quite right. He also came and sat in the orange tree to scold Mummy and drive her off before she stole any of his oranges.

I hope you are lucky enough to be able to enjoy your work as much as I do mine. It makes a great difference if you like your work. I liked school but not so much as I like work now.

* * *

I thought you would like a letter written by me looking down on the Amazon. (This sounds rather rude!) It is a thousand miles from its mouth. When I was small and we lived in Delhi we saw the Ganges (not from the air though, because the first aeroplane had not flown then!) and it was two miles wide 900 miles from the sea.

* * *

The Americans have any number of serious problems both international and private—starting with Vietnam and North Korea. But I am sure you realize the terrible lot that you have to learn which is *not* in the curriculum and cannot be taught by others though you have to learn it. You are fortunate, or rather *we* are, in that you seem able to learn about people and how you have to deal with them. This is fundamental no matter what you have to do by the way of life work. I feel that you will think I am preaching a sermon if I go on like this!

With all my love. We think of you all a great deal you may be sure.

* * *

The other day I was at a cross-roads watching the cars go by. They often have deep nasty dips at road intersections so if you go by at speed the car just about knocks you out—brains you, if you keep your brains in your bottom if you see what I mean. Well, car after car was going over this intersection and each one nearly rammed its chassis on to the road. This is a fault many of them have by having a soft suspension. Then suddenly one appeared and glided over with just a faint twinkle of its wheels as if it was giving me a wink—no prize offered for what the make was! There are two beauties—both brand new—which I see outside my office. American owned of course. I think it would take a very long time before I owned one. However, life has its compensations even if it does not include a Rolls Royce.

* * *

For heaven's sake don't turn into a bruiser! And don't get punch drunk or it will be goodbye to your A levels for ever. The boxer who owned Wells Rise before us could hardly tell if it was yesterday or tomorrow, but then he may not have been very bright even before anyone had beaten his face, skull and brains into a sort of batter pudding. Anyway—don't come back here looking like

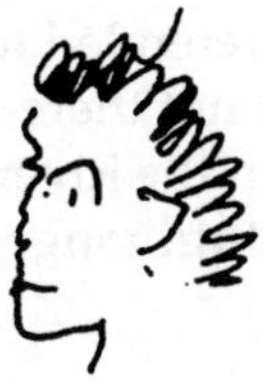

or

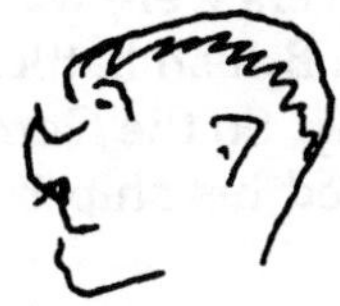

please!

Or they will spend so long looking through your stuff at customs that it will be time to go back before you've arrived. And keep your collar and tie on and you hair short. They are sure to be looking for drugs as all the smuggling here is done by school boys and girls and it makes them more suspicious still if you look like

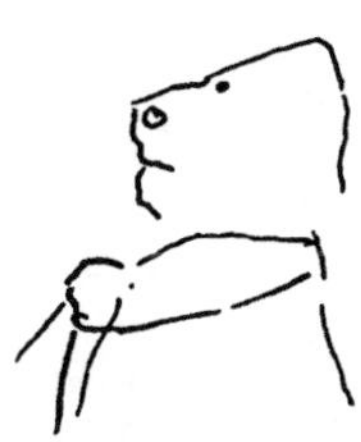

or

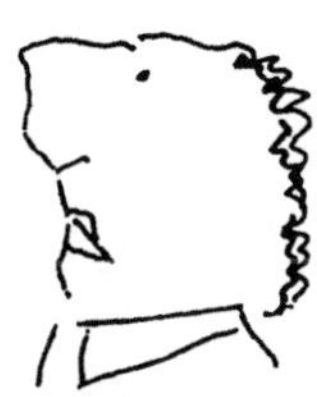

or

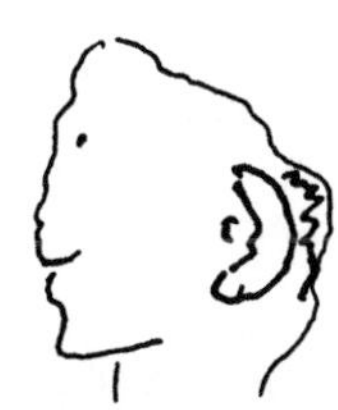

* * *

The Congreso National[1] (Parliament) is shut up because a dictator is running the country and he does not like parliaments. The River Plate (Rio de Plata) is so called because originally the early buccaneers came to Argentine for silver—that is why it is called Argent(ina). Similarly the River Plate is the river they went down to get 'plate'—hence silver or 'plate'. In the last war three small British ships chased a much bigger and faster German 'pocket' battleship, and though the Von Spee was supposed to be able to keep out of range and sink

[1] In Buenos Aires.

each one in turn without being hit, Commodore Harewood so ran the battle that one destroyer put down a smoke screen and the other one darted in and out of it, fired at the Von Spee and disappeared before the battleship could hit it. The British cruiser Essex got hit early and had to stop to repair its engine. So the two destroyers carried on alone and damaged the Von Spee so badly that it fled up the River Plate to Montevideo. When it finally had to come out the British destroyers were waiting for it and pretended to be signalling messages to a British battleship which was not there—it was about 900 miles away. So the Germans came down the River Plate and the captain scuttled his ship before getting within range of the British ships.

* * *

Last week-end Mummy and I went to a convention of psychoanalysts at San Diego. We did not have time to go to the zoo, the animal one I mean, which was a pity because it is world-famous. I was giving a paper to the human one. It was not very good but I got it done and that was a great relief.

1969

I am with Mummy at the pool edge in the sunlight. I have been living for a short time at the rate of about £10,000 a year—in other words enjoying smoking one of your birthday cigars. It makes me feel moral and opulent and like shaking my head solemnly and saying to you, 'Ah my child; whatever you do don't imitate your Dad! Above all—DON'T SMOKE CIGARS!' Unless of course you first take the precaution of having £10,000 a year.

* * *

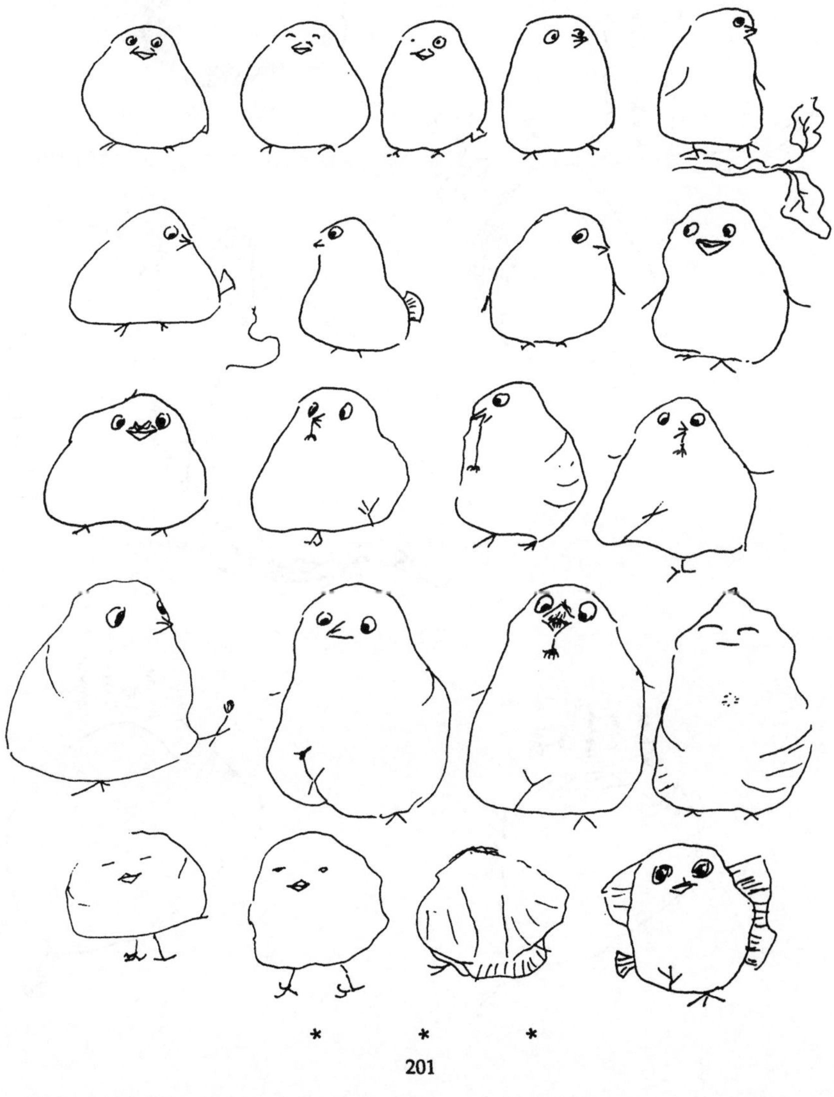

* * *

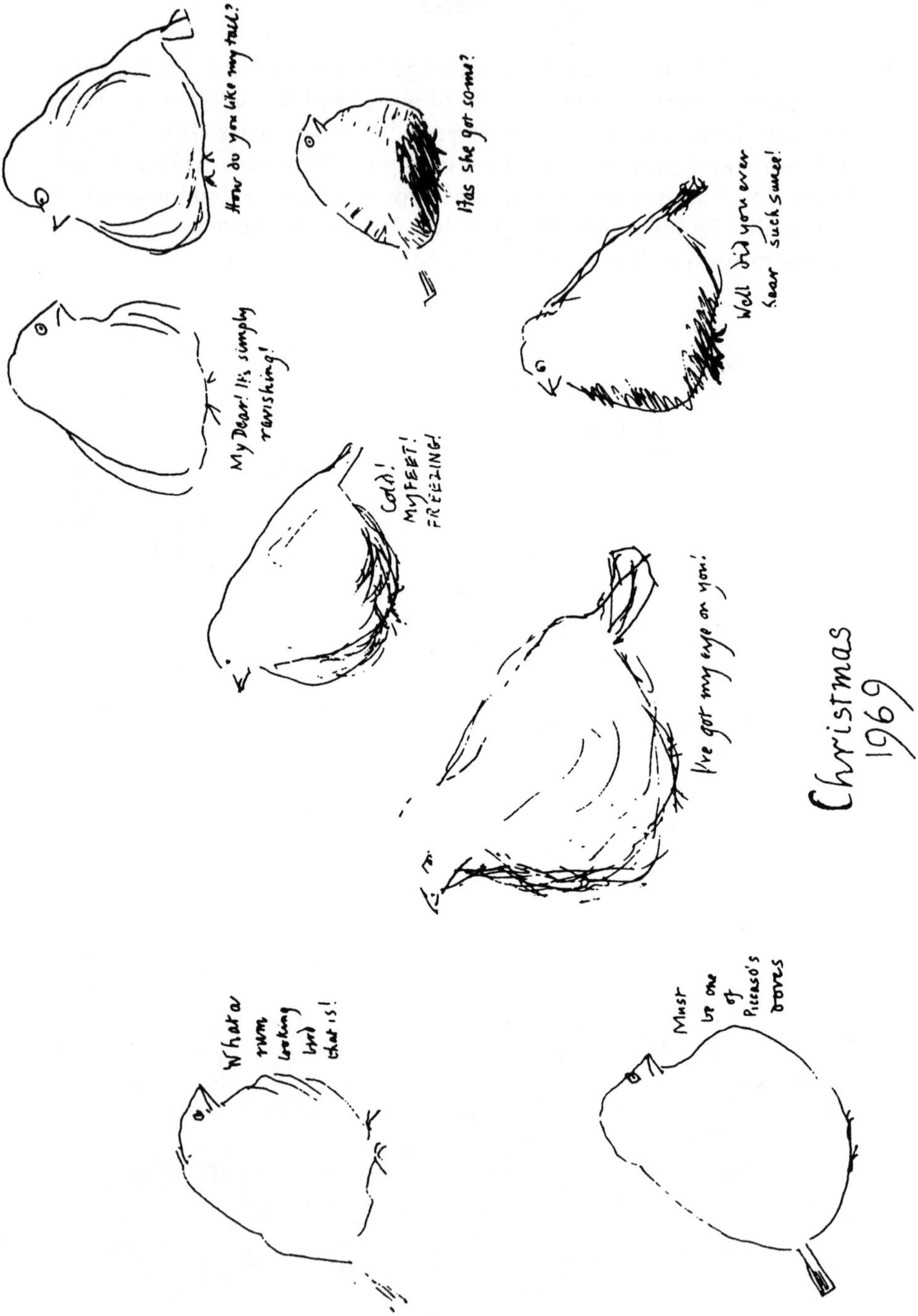
How do you like my tail?
Has she got some?
Well did you ever hear such swee!
My Dear! It's simply ravishing!
Cold! MY FEET! FREEZING!
I've got my eye on you!
Christmas 1969
What a rum looking bird that is!
Must be one of Picasso's doves

1970

It has become such a cliché that it is almost impossible to realize that in fact it is a great advantage if one gets the knack of 'making the best of things' however damn silly or worse the things are of which you are supposed to make the best. Life is a kind of Hoffnung's orchestra—if you have a bit of hosepipe and can use it as a French horn it is useful. Though I would not go so far as to suggest that if a fly sits on your music you should, like the short-sighted German, learn how to 'play 'eem'.

1971

There does not seem to be anything to do but start a letter and add instalments until such time as the posts start again, if ever.[1] We are bothered because of the chance—or certainty—of a railway strike.[2] When I was doing my medical training we had the General Strike and I was hoping to get round to driving a railway engine. But it all came to an end before I got that far. Just as well for me and any passengers who might have been so unlucky as to have me for their loco man. I hope it does not get as bad as that although, because that is nearer a revolution than a strike.[3]

* * *

We have just seen the Apollo blast-off on TV. ('If you've seen one blast-off you've seen them all'.) Sometimes it almost seems as if the moon may not be a bad place to be going to, but that I suppose is because there is no chance of being offered the trip.

"Cure", said our neurological chief, "is a gloomy subject—the only thing is that *our* patients don't die. All the others in medicine do." Not exactly a fair comment, but I can see what he meant. That is one reason I do not admit that psycho-analysis has really anything at all to do with cure. And now the other way round as well—cure has nowt to do with medicine.

As Mummy and I were sleeping the profound sleep of innocence there was suddenly a devilish and horrible noise. "There's that bloody picture down again", I thought angrily, determined not to be fooled again as I was last time when it nearly brained us and I thought it was an earthquake. Well, this time it wasn't the picture. Mummy dived to get under the bed—she couldn't, it is too low and there is no room. I took my usual precautions—got under the bed clothes. This scheme—of which I make a present to you—has always worked and is a sovereign cure and protection against mosquitoes, 5.9 howitzer shells, tigers, phosgene, mustard gas, bad dreams and earthquakes. You cannot always tell which is which when you are asleep and it's very useful to have something which is a cure for the lot. As I couldn't find the picture, and Mummy was behaving in such an unusual manner, I decided it must be a dream, but as I could not

[1] There was a postal strike in the U.K.
[2] In the U.K.
[3] In 1972 there was a coal strike in January, a railway strike in April, and a dock strike in August.

fall asleep it slowly became clear that it was no good trying to go on dreaming. We got up. By this time it was what passes for a fine sunny morning in these parts, so I was surprised to find it had apparently been raining very heavily. I pointed out this peculiar and interesting fact to Mummy. She, who seemed to be at least two days ahead of me, explained that it was the swimming pool which had slopped over. On the way down to the office she explained it was Tuesday and shortly after I more or less got the hang of the thing—rather like "*Can* curl but can't swim—swimming pool *that's* him".

The house, to my intense surprise, seems all right but I have no doubt that the roof will leak like a sieve when the heavy rains start which of course they are supposed to do any day soon. Lucky it wasn't already raining. In this district we have been extremely fortunate though some houses have some bad cracks. The worst, as you may have heard, is in the San Fernando Valley where the poor wretches in the Veterans Hospital got caught in the collapse of the building. Since then we have had a hundred or more 'temblors' as they call them—odd trembles, creaks and groans.

My attempts to reform my writing are not, as you can see, a success. I should have been taught to write when I was a child, but no one ever seemed to think that Public Schools should teach the children to write in return for the very high fees: even if they had, they would have taught copper-plate with all its curley-wigs I suppose. Anyway if one will not or cannot write properly it is no good blaming one's school or other people. You will never regret having started off on the right track because then I think you always have a fine hand even though you change it.

On Wednesday I gave my paper.[1] The majority of people who hate Kleinians did not come, but a few faithfuls came, as, to be quite fair, they would in England to show how bad and incomprehensible the paper was. I found it quite interesting but being an old hand at the job I was not surprised to find that even the eager supporters were *so* disappointed etc., etc., etc. So I think it must have been up to the usual standard. If the criticism is too laudatory I think one needs to become suspicious. You will have to get used to the idea that if you don't satisfy or, if you are fortunate, please yourself, you won't please anyone else.

* * *

[1] 'The Grid'.

We look forward to hearing about your holiday. You will have seen it before it disappears beneath masses of tourists, atom bombs and such like disasters. I alas have never been to Greece. I think Plato's Socratic Dialogues would have meant even more to me than they did if I had been able to imagine the background: and heaven knows it was a revelation as it was. Perhaps because I read them at the right time when Oxford was opening my mind to the pleasures of philosophy.

* * *

I spent most of my time as a medico feeling that another week of it and I should go nuts. Anyhow if you survive to pass Anatomy and Physiology you can reckon you can survive almost anything—though I have known contemporaries of mine who reckoned 'Midder'[1] to run Urogenital Firm very close as being rock bottom (or anyhow, 'bottom').

* * *

Here we are in Mexico City. We took plane on Monday, everyone being really worn out. It is *not* a satisfactory state to be in before a holiday though I suppose one can argue that it is at least better before than after. I feel like a piece of chewed string; I haven't a mind—just a hardened mass of congealed clichés which have become stuck together. As I become aware of my surroundings, it might be Europe. Here, with a population of a mere couple of million indigent poor, they have a book shop every hundred yards or so. In Beverly Hills there are two well-stocked book shops and a branch elsewhere. If you ask for a book they haven't got they seem to think, hopefully, that another one will do—just like, but really rather better; e.g. Q. Have you *The Gemstones of Southern California?* A. No-o-o. Here's one—*The Stones of Venice*—would that do?" Q. No: it's not Venice down by Culver City—Venice in Italy, you know." A. Oh—it's by Ruskin who is said to be a good author. I haven't read it myself." Resisting the temptation to say, "I can see that", one passes on.

[1] Midwifery.

1972

As you can imagine, Mummy and I read any scraps we can get from you and friends and others—even from papers—about what is going on.[1] The only thing we can be *sure* of discovering is that we *don't* know, can't know and never shall know. I once—I am talking about the first war—felt sure that at the end I should know, if I was still in existence, who had won. Well, I know that I *don't* know, but I *think* I know we did *not*. Even *that* I am not sure of; you can see it depends where you write FINIS; the end of the first day of the Cambrai battle? End of first week, month, year? Century perhaps? You see how complicated a simple question like, 'Who won the Battle of Cambrai?' turns out to be. Anyhow, you and others must be damned cold—with the fear of being colder still if it is not possible to earn a living or get anyone else to do it for us.

It is now 11.0 a.m. on Sunday. Mummy and I are sitting by the pool. Temperature is 60° in the shade but we are in the sun which is very warm. I tell you this as a contrast to what you must be having—pity you can't prop this up against the wall and warm your hands at it. Even if it made you hot with envy it would be something, but I am afraid it is not even that much use. It certainly wasn't when—rarely—I was sitting about shivering in a trench consoling myself that if I got warm the lice would start biting.

* * *

All these problems are demanding solution all over the world, only in different stages of development. It is like the state in the Universe where, if you had the skill and the technical equipment—and lots of equipment you cannot even guess at—you could know a great deal about everything from man and his so-called mind, to quasars and other animals not even available to us for inspection in our present state of 'blissful' ignorance. Oh for the days (Past/Future) which (were/will be) the Ones! There's also a lot to be said for being able to live—where one has to anyway—in the present.

* * *

You will have heard from Mummy of my various medical capers: so now I write you of certain physiological aspects—clinical I should rather say—which I find quite interesting.

[1] During the coal strike in the U.K.

It started on a Monday morning with my not feeling too good and not feeling so bad either. Then with my midday patient I couldn't think very clearly which I did not bother about as the patient pours it out non-stop and I didn't feel it was much out of the ordinary. *Then* I felt my right arm wouldn't work and began trying to find out—while listening to the patient—if I had had a stroke. But it didn't seem to be a hemiplegic. It was now the end of the session and I dared not get out of my chair, in case I could not, and I did not want it poured out to all my patients that I had had a 'stroke'. So, picking out what seemed least likely to cause the greatest trouble I stayed put and excused myself for not rising at his departure. He seemed a bit surprised but he left. I could pull myself together enough to bring the next one in and tell him I wuld have to cancel. He seemed a bit surprised but cleared off. Both of them then rang up within the next twenty minutes to find out if I was OK which seemed very decent. In the meantime the landlord at my request brought a Dr D. and he set me to cancel all my other patients and to fill in four sheets of forms. I would have liked samples of them to send you because they seemed to be a very good idea and one which would pretty well make it certain that the doctor had examined all systems. It struck me how very useful it would be now, and certainly later, to draw up your own private questionnaire and so make sure that you never missed anything of importance when it came to examining a patient. My greatest triumph in that way was to get a gold medal for senior clinical surgery by saying, when asked to examine and describe a swelling of the knee joint, that I would not give a definite diagnosis until I had had an X-ray of the chest! Quite right of course! You might as well work out what the anatomy of the chest has got to do with the anatomy of the knee-joint. Anyway the result was a perfectly good Gold Medal. I must have known something else too but I have no memory of it. I think that itself suggests gold medals must be very bad for surgery.

Now D. did apply his stethoscope and his knee hammer, and he did say he wanted me to go into hospital to be thoroughly tested. This fearsome prospect I resisted, like a fool, As it turned out he, also like a fool, let me have my way. I say 'like a fool' but I am not sure that it would not have been even more foolish to have insisted and raised my anxiety to catastrophic heights. It may indeed have been wiser to let me go my own way. By putting me on immediate sodium-free diet (ghastly!! but I have now got used to it, more or less) and extra potassium, I felt miles better at the end of the week. But I 'co-operated' so much that the whole process of reduction was too violent. Result: Tuesday—suddenly lost consciousness and when I recovered I was under Dr S. in Midway Hospital. This time, I'm bound to admit, very much to my relief and too ill even to think, let alone worry, about finance. What poor Mummy had to put up with I leave you to imagine—I can't. Anyway, after a week of 'Intensive Care', on Monday morning back home again I came and tomorrow I see S. again. I am to get my weight down to 164 lbs; I have so far gone from 196 to 184 lbs.

'Intensive care' nursing—ludicrous. Sheets never smoothed out but left hideously uncomfortable and, as likely as not, not covering one. Thermometer left in ten or more minutes. Urine bottles, bed pans etc. left under patient sometimes for half an hour or more. Chat between nurses, loud, at any hour of day and night, and patients unable to get care unless insisting on it.

All mechanical tests good, expensive and efficient. The nearer they get medicine to computer medicine, and that is the way to go and the way they are going, the sooner they will leave the rest of the world out of sight. In so far as doctors, the best of them, have to be capable of compassion for human beings who are suffering, the more bleak the outlook. It was pathetic to see how nurses, and for that matter some subordinate doctors, responded to some sign of interest in their affairs. The ideal of course would be if one could respect people *and* respect the truth (facts).

* * *

The news of the end of the strike was a great relief to us though it is anything but a relief to understand, especially for *this* psychoanalyst, why our country should have to be ruined before a commission could be caused to do some thinking. What is a Coal Board for? What are trade unions and their leaders for? What are governments for? But of course they are the all-wisest as well as the All-Highest; such things are too deep for me, and it is, I suppose, as well that I have to do an insignificant job and just die quietly of bad temper! Still, I don't see why you should be burdened with this tirade. I have enough sense—just—to know it's not your fault.

* * *

The whole of my letter looks remarkably ill-written compared with your written script. In my time, that any *man* would bother to have good writing manners would have been unthinkable and as a result the products of the so-called public schools were a lot of uncivil unlettered boors without even a suspicion that this might be so. You have the fortunate chance that you may always write an easy, beautiful and civilized letter.

* * *

I have been on a diet of 1 gram of sodium and 1200 calories a day. With this I have potassium three times a day and cyclospasmol 100gm and I think I feel better than I have at any time since I came to the U.S. I am to get my weight down to 12 stone—which is quite something, but I have so far gone from 14 stone to 13st 2lbs. I am starving and unfortunately Mummy feels obliged to be similarly starved in sympathy. But for me it is a very good thing and therefore no hardship; not so for her.

The Times Lit. Supp., which thinks it is the World's Most Famous Journal of the kind, would not publish a letter of mine. OK! But they wrote a routine would-be 'polite' letter of rejection, and showed their immense superiority to me by being 'very interested' but failing to realize I was a doctor—*printed* heading notwithstanding—and got my name wrong too! 'Incompetent, Slovenly, Snooty': our version of 'Liberty, Equality, Fraternity', when we finally succeed in staying out of the Common Market.

* * *

Sorry about the boredom of the course. You have to learn what to do with boredom and bores—Pope had his method in writing, itself an antidote, and describing the bores in *The Dunciad:* let me lend you my copy when you are back here. Bores and boredom are never in short supply—dieters, so-self-called exponents of 'dietary' exercise and their very close cousins who slim are a not inconsiderable part of that vast Mississippi with great megatons of boredom floating around in it. Good luck in your navigation of that 'fascinating' stream. Sorry I can't do more than wish you well.

With regard to the Pharmacology book—'excellence' has to be paid for: never get anything less. As I have said before, 'Get it or go without' till you *can* get it. Don't buy rubbish: rubbish is *expensive at any price.* Get the Pharmacology and keep it—i.e. don't let anyone borrow or steal it. Never lend books—all borrowers are thieves whatever they say, no matter how rich or respectable. *Our* riches and respectability are of course always vulnerable to attack by anyone who feels disposed to destroy either our financial assets or our reputation for integrity and reliability.

Keep fit: 'Bored but buoyant' be the watchword so that you remain afloat, if possible.

* * *

In The Listener I see there is a long article on the great Ronnie Laing. I had him taking up one of my seminars to psycho-analytic students, teaching me all about it—he still not then being qualified. So his self-appointed importance is nothing new. The article ends with his having gone into a Cingalese monastery. Good idea! Very wise, and I would not sometimes mind a dose of the same medicine myself.

* * *

It is curious to see how little they seem even to understand the biology of the so-called hallucinogenic drugs today. It looks as if the Royal Court at Ur used the ritualistic function of—hashish?—on entry into the Death Pit. The remnants of the Aztec religion, still very much alive, is well and truly established in the Native American Church; they have, despite the efforts of the R.C. Church, been able to win their case in the U.S. Supreme Court allowing them the continued use of hallucinogenic drugs for sacramental and ritualistic purposes.

* * *

We went on the beach this morning for about an hour. People 'fishing', if that's what you call it and don't get it confused with 'catching fish'. For that it is better to go to a fishmonger. I caught a trout once but it must have been daft.

* * *

My shoes still look brand new although they are maturing beautifully. Of course I don't walk on them, and cannot now say I even use them for the accelerator and brake. Finally I suppose feet will become vestiges (in America) and no more use than the tail. There ought to be a medical course in Vestigiology to match Embryology.

* * *

It was a most unfortunate accident.[1] Mummy called an ambulance. Arrangements were then made that Dr W. would wait for me at Cedars Sinai Hospital. I was taken to, and waited at Cedars Sinai. No one had heard of what I was doing hanging around Cedars Sinai and cluttering up the works. I said, "X-ray of hip—Dr W." Answer: Never heard of him. You must have doctor's authority. Ambulance said, "Oh sorry—wrong hospital!—about twenty miles further from home. "Too late—too bad—can't change now!. "Dr M. will see you". The X-ray could then take over, bored to death with the body they hadn't asked anyone for. Keeping my views to myself and apologizing profusely for my existence (I should DAMN WELL THINK SO!), had a spinal general anaesthetic and ultimately found myself in bed. Luckily too anaesthetized to know more than the hellish cold and stayed put till about 9.30 a.m. Mummy was told by a Dr E. that he had operated on me. "All well."

Last Wednesday morning I was booted out back home—Mummy I need hardly say has been miraculous although with merely human equipment to do it.

[1] Carrying his painting easel in the garden, he tripped and fell, fracturing his right femur.

1973

The thing I am supposed to be writing, thanks to Mummy's efforts, is I think about done.[1] It seems pretty unreadable to me but I hope it's not as bad as it seems. I cannot say I feel any real hope about getting it published, let alone sold after that. The one book that I couldn't be bothered with, even when pressure was put on me ten years later, has been a continuous success.[2] But writing books is no way of making a living—that's clear.

If you are to get a job you will have to fight for it—nature red in tooth and claw. All the other claws and teeth will be in good working order too. In England just as much as here; here just as much as there. In fun as well as in fight. Even in love claws and teeth are out—in action, I don't mean 'ruled out'. Stalin was asked if he would support the English Communists. "Yes!" he said, and then added, "As much as a rope supports a man who is hanged". Franco said much the same about how he would show his gratitude for the help that the Nazis had given him. "When I have won", he said, "the world will be amazed at my display—of gratitude of course." Someone thought he winked but it may have been a speck of dust.

* * *

We were glad to hear that you are finding the medical course more interesting now you have got on to the clinical stuff. I often wish I had made more use of it when I had a chance. I was not in fact very bright and had my mind too much fixed on psychological stuff to see my chance to do quite a lot of things which I might have been doing with a less one-track mind. However, regretting one's misspent youth is a very easy way of mis-spending *other* opportunities and is extremely boring as well. So I will desist.

* * *

The Brazil visit went off very well and was enjoyable and rewarding.[3] They want me to go again in December or later. People here also want me to stay here—or so they think. It sounds like someone's description of a second marriage as an example of Hope triumphing over Experience.

* * *

[1] *A Memoir of the Future*, Book I, *The Dream*. Imago Editora. Rio de Janeiro, 1975. *see also* p.222.
[2] *Experiences in Groups*, Tavistock Publications, 1961.
[3] Two weeks of seminars and lectures in São Paulo.

The drug I use for my 'arteries' is called Cyclospasmol. Its action is to decoke the arteries, allowing the blood, if any, unobstructed flow. Contra indications—if it is bad for you. Good for: ingrowing toenails, unwanted hair on the face, schizophrenia of course, tsutsugumachie fever, boredom, yaws and beriberi. Bio-chemistry—doesn't do a damn thing but is harmless; luckily its effects wear off very quickly and any obstruction that has itself been temporarily obstructed, soon re-establishes itself. As far as I am concerned I await, without anxiety or interest, the discovery that it causes various diseases. As Walsh, our neurological chief, used to say, "Medicine is *not* an art; it is *not* a science; it is a sport". To which I would add, it is also an addiction and can occasionally cause dangerous side-effects. As another of my chiefs—Bernard Hart—said on one occasion after he had listened carefully to a psychiatric social worker introducing the new patient, "Ah . . .", looking up cautiously at the end of the long tirade, "and which is the nurse and which is the patient?" I am sure I have told you this before, but there is nothing wrong with me: old age is not a disease, but people—bless their hearts—long to cure one. But one has to exercise a certain caution lest they kill you off in the process. So far I have survived.

* * *

I never argue against other people's views. They (1) don't pay any attention, (2) use it to prove you are wrong, (3) get downright nasty about it and never forgive you, (4) pinch your idea when they have found out what it is, or (3) and (4). Only read the best—e.g. Freud and Klein: and acknowledge what you take. Acknowledging a bad writer is like becoming responsible for, *and* advertising him. You can see from the foregoing what a nasty character I have; alas, one does not improve with age.

* * *

I usually feel in this queer job of mine that I have hardly anything to say from the depths in other people's unconscious, and by the time I have emerged from that into the 'glare' of other people's conscious I am too blindly bat-like to have anything to say.

* * *

Gerald Brenan has been translating—I don't know how well, but he should be good—Saint John of the Cross, his mystical poems. I think you probably remember Roy Campbell's efforts. He should have been good, but without knowing any Spanish and relying only on what I know of Saint John's mysticism, it seemed to me that the translations sounded a bit as if they were off the wave length—not quite sympathetic to that type of mind.

Gilbert and Sullivan *and* concerts *and* plays—well it's a bust eight weeks even if you do try to cram in a degree during your spare time. I am sure I am very bad to speak so disrespectfully of serious things, but perhaps you will re-interpret my letter in suitably gloomy terms and take it as 'understood' even if not exactly stated that life is serious, gloomy and earnest, d—— it!

* * *

Poor Rupert Brooke! I always liked his poetry though now I gather that if anyone reads, 'If I should die, think only this of me —', they mutter to themselves, "You did, and we don't —" Perhaps this is an exaggeration.

Congratulations on finding *Sesame and Lilies* — *and* being able to enjoy it. I have always had a soft spot for Ruskin. Complete works, beautiful paper and print in Sothern's — price? £500! Even now probably worth buying, but 500 worthless pounds take an awful lot of hard work to earn.

* * *

Here they are making much of the Lambton case[1] to show that the British are as bad [as those involved in the Watergate scandal]. I must say the British being morally horror struck about sex is a ludicrous and ultimately nauseating spectacle. But Jellicoe and Lambton must indeed be peculiar people to choose for goverment position—they should find grown-ups (of whatever age) for jobs of that kind.

* * *

Poor Flavio de Carvalho has died—the man who painted the portrait of me in São Paulo.Although only having met him for a few hours I liked him—we both did, very much. I think he was gifted—

[1] The disappearance of Lord Lambton who was never seen again.

maybe much more—and both Mummy and I like the portrait, both as a painting and a likeness, though I think that most people would dislike it. I am no beauty and no one seeing this would suppose I was. However, I am not wanting to advertise 'beauty aids' so that's all right. When it dries off, by the end of the year I think, it can be varnished and framed.

* * *

I do not know Rio but from what we hear of it we both like the *prospect*. The reality of the far-off hills at closer inspection can turn out to be different. The situation here is one of such suspicion—and who can blame them!—that it is hardly possible either to have *any* interpretation respected because an ulterior is suspected as the real motive, or not to dread the patient's mental apparatus.

* * *

One would be very foolish to imagine that people (all of them) are very different when one looks into it closely—which of course is precisely what one is supposed to do. Here they have had to bow, be it never so unwillingly, to the fact that, when one gets past the ridiculous hate and messianic adulation, one has *some* experience if they can bear to admit it. Then one gets into the more steady and more nearly permanent state of envy and robbery, or merely theft. Here, as at Buenos Aires, I am now admitted to know something but am so unable to express myself that others do it far better and are better suited to lecturing. Still, as I haven't the time, wish or drive I cannot really complain and I don't wish to sink into a grizzly and miserable old age of feeling 'ill-treated'. That is a truly ungenerous state of mind, an insult to the Almighty when I consider that I have always been one of the pampered and privileged classes. Luckily Mummy knows that even better than I do.

* * *

My memories of the Varsity were in far more rigid days and we were, as I see it now, a pretty battered crowd of psychological wrecks just out of the war. I remember thinking Queen's dons were a bit soft in the head because they did not expect much from us; 'they (us) couldn't be expected to do very well after the strain of war'. Now I realize of course they were quite right. In the last war (Great, second lap) they didn't allow youngsters to get into fighting but *I* was only almost twenty-one at the *end* of my fighting career and I have since only very slowly come to realize what a *very* long time it took me to recover. I hope you have none of that kind of thing to put up with and that England manages to keep out of *that* sort of trouble now we aren't supposed to be of any importance compared with the 'super-powers', U.S. and Russia. Not glorious, maybe, but let us hope a chance to rediscover our greatness as a civilization. Goodness knows the burden this small country has tried to carry as the world's leading nation—it has just about sucked us dry and bankrupt in every way. But now of course we are liable to attack by the bullies and blackguards who cannot resist the temptation of the weak and helpless.

1974

I seem to spend many hours doing 'nothing' unless you count reading books, but even so they often seem to come to 'nothing' because they turn out to be irrelevant but good, or worse still, bad but irrelevant. Then some are irrelevant but interesting. A few are irrelevant, uninteresting *and* bad, and *they* are usually compulsory reading. I hope this is not your fate though I must say that the time I spent in France as a 'student' was utterly wasted by me. But probably it was because I was not happy at that time, wondering—as I still am—how on earth to earn enough money. But I have at least the consolation of feeling there is nothing more likely to make it possible than knowing one's job. The snag is that one never seems to feel one knows one's job. Luckily, if you have the guts to dare to believe it, enjoying one's job is a very good indicator.

When I was in Tours about 1921, I went into a bookshop and Anatole France was sitting in a chair in the corner. A Frenchman came in, looked at him and tapped his own forehead in a knowing way. Indicating Anatole France, he said to the shopkeeper, "Voilà un type idiot!' and walked out. France was amused—but not I think flattered!

In a fortnight we leave for Brazil. The work will be a change though I find myself wondering what on earth I shall have to tell them. One day I shall stand in front of my audience and goggle at them helplessly—lecturer's nightmare—especially since I always leave it till the occasion to say what I am going to say instead of preparing. Once I was told I sounded unprepared, to which I replied, "That's quite true—if you leave out the preceding 70 years".

* * *

Never lose the flair for coping with

1. not enough time
2. not enough knowledge
3. not the proper conditions
4. sick and disturbed patients *and* sick and disturbed doctors, chiefs and colleagues as well.

All these four are essential ingredients if you are having *real* medicine in *real* life, and to hell with what the text books *say* it is. Incidentally I see some bright spark is saying that Onassis hasn't got myasthenia gravis because he's got a deep form of influenza which is affecting his capacity to breathe!!! I remember warning a doctor who sent me a neurotic patient; I tried to tell him firmly but gently that he had myesthenia gravis and I was afraid that terminal weakness of the thoracic muscles would set in and lead to his death through respiratory failure if this were not immediately treated. He wrote to me a week or so later to say I was mistaken and that the patient had died through an attack of 'flu which had become pneumonia despite his care. I wonder that we survive when you consider how wrong, ignorant, and mistaken we psycho-analysts are! The trouble you are having is familiar, so you may as well get hardened to it—if you are tough enough to survive—*now.* I think I was lucky to survive two wars. Now of course I only have to cope with Peace. We have to learn to carry on our peaceable avocations amidst the warring states of the Modern Dark Ages.

* * *

I think it is high time for the good of the world that Europe was re-constituted. And Ireland rowed out to sea and sunk. It annoys me to feel that our troops have to continue to be embroiled.

* * *

I am not surprised that psychiatry has been a bit disillusioning—so is psycho-analysis or virtually any human activity, because for some reason when 'mind meets mind', or 'boy meets girl', or 'boy meets boy', or 'X meets Y', they shy off it as if shot and one begins to feel it is dangerous to like one's own kind. So it is. But—not all *that* dangerous. However, whether it is physical medicine, or psychological 'medicine', or not any kind of medicine, two people seem to find it very difficult to do, and psychiatrists and psycho-analysts are as bad (worse?) than the rest. Anyhow, you may learn how *not* to do it and that is after all quite a valuable lesson.

Brazil was stimulating to me. I often feel I could learn a lot—'had I —. .' etc. etc. Truman wisely says never waste time on regret.[1] In Rio a woman turned up on hearing of our presence and introduced herself to Mummy. She, it appears, is a Bion having a grandfather called Gabriel from Bordeaux who came from La Rochelle. Our Huguenot ancestors also came from there, via Switzerland, St Gall, and England, so it seems more than likely there are Brazilian Bions as well. Up the clan!

* * *

[1] *Plain Speaking: An Oral Biography of Harry S. Truman*, Merle Miller, Berkley Publishing Corp., 1974.

I hope you are able to squeeze in a bit of medicine in your spare time—without of course going so far as actually catching the complaints. Being a chef may of course turn out to be far more profitable if there is anything to cook. France can actually export food, which is far from the case with England who may therefore have to export people. So far I myself seem to have a certain sale value but one never knows—and never knew—how long that will last.

I appear to retain outrageously good health chiefly, it sometimes seems, through 'eating that which I ought not to have eaten'. I don't recommend you to follow in my teeth marks. Goodbye and 'cueillez dès aujourd'hui les roses de la vie',[1] or as Voltaire has it, 'cultivez votre jardin'. By the way, get hold of Voltaire's *Candide*—it's slap up to date.

* * *

Time rushes by, so it won't be long before you are off to Vietnam. We have no idea of how much we shall be able to hear of you or to keep in touch with you, or what sort of experience you will have. Of course I remember launching out—at long last it seemed—to France and war. Now I realize that those were relatively civilized days although incredibly lethal. So you are probably in for something which will vary from the utterly banal—days, weeks, one hopes not years, of 'nothing'—to times of intense danger. Usually it changes from utter boredom to utter horror without any warning and apparently no transition from one to the other. Do not imagine that anyone *loves* you—and do not be surprised into taking it as a personal grievance when you find they *don't!*

This place thinks a recession is coming and I don't doubt it or believe it. We *think* we shall be asked to Brasilia and that we shall probably get there, but I find it hard nowadays to be particularly impressed by my own or anybody else's foresight. "Vivez, si m'en croyez —".[1] I still have an inner impulse to do a bit more roving even at my decrepit, but not more discreet, old age. There is, I fear, no fool quite like an *old* fool. But Brasilia is rather nice don't you think? Perhaps only when separated by a waste of seas. I am also attracted by the fact of a sprig of the La Rochelle branch (of the family) being in Rio.

It is a great comfort to be able to feel that, so far, you all survive. It is incredible how little one can do for one's own family, and how much each one has to learn to do for him or her self. That is why a

[1] Ronsard, 'Sonnets pour Hélène', Bk. 2, XIII.

husband or wife is so important—the only person one can ever hope to meet who will augment such slender capacity as the 'one' alone is lucky to have.

* * *

Many thanks for your birthday card and good wishes—I'm sorry you seem to have been so disturbed by having forgotten it. I doubt people of 77 should really set much store about whether we do or do not have another to add to the store of spent or mis-spent birthdays! Here I had a fine birthday cake and found that my taste for it remains in unabated health and vigour; must have the secret of perpetual youth as do all my other reprehensible and uninteresting characteristics.

* * *

As far as exams are concerned, the important thing is to get used to them! Exam-passing has not got much to do with the subject, but has a lot to do with 'passing exams'. The examiners usually know that even the best scholars write a lot of damned nonsense anyway. They *try*, that is the examiners try, especially in Finals to get people to stop and think, if possible *after* reading the questions, *before* writing anything. If by some fluke you seem to have written sense don't let it go to your head but just plug on steadily.

P.S. It is of course useful, even in exams, but not essential, to know the *subject*—*if* you can keep you head and remember you are supposed to be *passing*. But don't get confused and make the mistake of thinking that exam-passing and knowing French or Chinese or Sanskrit is the same thing, or that if you (or even a don) have passed an exam you really know the subject. You *may*, but it is not necessarily true. Going to a good university is a chance of becoming *wiser* by the time you leave, but that is not included in the schedule. You can always mug up what is in the schedule; but becoming wiser is nothing to do with 'swotting' and you may be *becoming* wiser in your sleep.

Learn either Russian or Chinese or Sanskrit provided you don't let it interfere with becoming wiser by wanting to pass exams; that can be as bad as taking to drink or any other drug. Many a good man or woman has ruined themselves or their families by taking to drink; it is not so spectacular but just as ruinous to 'take to exam-passing'.

* * *

Alas, to think I wasted my time swimming at Oxford. As almost the only person in Oxford who could swim I had to captain it, collect a few of my contemporary unemployed rugger blues and teach them to tread water so they could represent Oxford against Cambridge without sinking to the bottom before the 'match'[1] was over, and then let these thugs loose against your U. on THE DAY. I used to swim around while my thugs quietly strangled your thugs in various quiet out-of-the-way spots in the Bath Club bath without the referee seeing what was going on. *But* we had a marvellous dinner afterwards and very amusing speeches. Poor old Lord Desborough used to be the chairman, a man whom I liked very much but with a family who all formed part of a real tragedy—not one of his sons was left before I had finished with Oxford. Still—not such a ghastly tragedy as we are able to witness with the Randolph Hearst family picking its way along the (American) primrose path. Who would be a multi-millionaire on those terms?[2]

My idiotic book has not been published yet, so such dregs of reputation as I still retain remain intact. I fear it might not survive publication—if that ever occurred.[3]

* * *

People here are very gloomy about the prospects financial and otherwise. It sounds queer for the wealthiest nation in the world but they 'know' and I don't think they are wrong. In 1906 when I first went to school, King George was saying,[4] "Wake up, England!" but alas, they didn't.

[1] Water polo.
[2] The daughter, Patricia, was kidnapped and subsequently took part in an armed bank robbery—whether voluntarily or by coercion remained unclear.
[3] *A Memoir of the Future*, Book I, *The Dream*.
[4] In 1901, when he was Prince of Wales.

1975

We were relieved to hear that you were back in London—safe, as we laughably imagine, for a moment or two though I have no doubt you will be off again shortly on further explorations. Not that I personally think one would ever be so foolish to imagine that anyone was safe anywhere, and though medicine—or an aim to help in any way—would ensure a certain welcome, in fact of course people *hate* being helped. Unless of course it gives them a chance to 'help' themselves, preferably to the helper's goods—watch, stethoscope, camera, and even ideas if they can. At school we always preferred to rob the orchard of a professional apple grower than help ourselves to the windfalls of a generous farmer who allowed us to collect what we liked by invitation.

I used to be *taught*, but never learned, that what you did with money was save it. Your Auntie Edna was infinitely more sensible so she has a home of her own but has a nasty character—don't tell her. I have a beautiful nature but *no* cash. There is a moral in all this I am sure . . .

I hope you persuade someone to 'qualify' you soon as it can be quite useful. So, I find, can *not* being qualified: it is a bit anxiety-provoking but on the other hand it saves one the danger of thinking that somone loves us and is anxious for us to survive. There is a nice story of C. E. Montague's in which he tells of a beetle that was almost caught by a tortoise and had the bright idea of scuttling into the pursuer's carapace in which he remained secure waiting for better times. 'Beneath the shadow of Thy wing Thy saints have dwelt secure' is a hymn we used to sing; but I have only just thought of this possible in-security.

I have been mugging up the pharmacology of porphyrin—very appropriate to these times. Maybe it applies to Vietnam and wisdom to know whether to back the Vietcong or the U.S. The Great Powers, 'Slow and solid that's him'—can't curl but can swim—or 'Stickly Prickly.[1]

However, 'good luck', provided you don't believe in it. The safest horse to bet on, believe it or not, is yourself.

* * *

[1] 'The Beginning of the Armadilloes', *Just So Stories*, Rudyard Kipling.

It is hard to believe that the world has to be governed by mere human beings. Now, thanks to nuclear fission they can *really* do some damage, whereas in the old days they could only damage people they could reach with a battle axe. "Saul has killed his thousands —", but nowadays we have even put David and his tens of thousands into the shade. Well, some fool will let off an atom bomb one day soon now, so we may as well make the best of our last days of human supremacy before we follow the dinosaurs into the shade. As we used to say in the days of World War I, "Don't forget to take a clean handkerchief in your pocket, and above all don't get your feet wet." (Advice before going into the line at Ypres.) Anyhow, although *you* may be disappointed, *we* don't want you to have any of that.

* * *

We have just been listening to Nixon on the State of the Nation. The speech—which one must call able and effective—was rapturously received; 'standing ovation' seems to be the normal form. It was Pie In The Sky writ large. The glorious 'feats of arms' and so on in Vietnam and after—it almost sounds as if the facts are of no consequence when served up with lots and lots of artificial butter, and indeed *that* I think is what analysis has to be here. I sincerely hope that in your experience of medicine you have enough of the luxury of doing a job honestly to develop a taste for it before your palate is irretrievably ruined.

The news from England is depressing including the apparently impenetrable optimism which it seems can withstand any fact that might be fired at *that* form of armour plate.

* * *

When you sit staring blankly and with sinking heart, and as all your mis-spent youth flashes like a horror movie before your eyes, try to read the exam paper through the distorting mirror of your scalding tears of misery and contrition, and you may notice some dregs of what you think is medicine. If so, with due circumspection, write it down; you may get a good mark or two and scrape through. Knowing medicine is very useful and not a positive hindrance to being qualified, *but* passing a medical exam is quite another business, or passing *any* exam. Don't afterwards find out how brilliantly everyone has done at the 'marvellous' paper. That way lies drink and a pauper's grave. I still scrape a living, but I could not for the life of me pass an exam in psycho-analysis, medicine, or any other subject. When I took 'Fevers' I could only think of tsusugemushi fever and then only because it reminded me of playing trains. The French in their queer way call it a 'teuf-teuf'. That was the first suspicion I had of the French who did not even know if *should* be 'puff-puff'.

* * *

I have been reading your Vietnam diary. I think you will find it very fortunate that you wrote so fully at the time it was fresh in your mind. I have only got half way through so far—I of course interpret what you write very much in terms of a battle front not so far away even though your job was a different kind of battle—disease. One cannot help being very moved by the sturdiness and courage of the children. I wish I could believe that they could rely on the 'grown-ups' being as wise or as sturdy. Alas, I don't.

* * *

I have finished reading Wavell's Memoirs. I never met him though I liked his son, Lord Karen, 'Archie', very much indeed. Wavell was the finest and most cultivated soldier we had, even greater than *his* hero, Allenby, I think. And what a raw deal he had, not least from Churchill I regret to say. But Churchill himself had a raw deal and was only given his chance when the riff-raff had lost the British Empire and wanted to have the dregs salvaged. "Pass it on!" we used to say in my prep school after punching our neighbour in the guts. *Very* funny, as you can see.

* * *

Apropos the Common Market, a story in the Manchester Guardian of a woman living in Streatham: when asked her opinion of the Common Market she replied, "I didn't know there was a market on the Common". A very sensible reply I think. In my time I hardly noticed Streatham Common when I was taking the dog for a walk. (Big enough for *his* purposes though!)

* * *

Yeats I met before the First War, and after it I remember his saying, with Aldous Huxley and George Moore, "What a pity they can't *all* be beaten!" Well, now it seems pretty clear that they *all* were. Perhaps we shall recover but that would not be an advantage if it were simply to be able to get back to the status quo.

* * *

The English summer seems, like us, to have come to California. It is cold and dark (or we have become so soft that we do not appreciate June in California).

> 'Thus may a captive in some fortress grim
> From casual speech betwixt his warders learn
> That June on her triumphal progress goes
> Through arched and bannered woodlands; while for him
> She is a legend emptied of concern.
> And idle is the rumour of the rose.'[1]

* * *

I gave a talk to the Research Committee—so called—though I was given the most dire warnings about the ranks of Midian (Gideon?). Yet it turned out all right. Two hundred nearer than the twenty I was given to expect, and as quiet as mice when the cat is around. For which I was truly thankful. I hate boisterous and hostile audiences and don't feel at all inclined to be helpful.

So—we are *in* the Common Market. Heaven's morning breaks and Earth's vain shadows flee (or not as the case may be).

* * *

The discovery that you have a MIND is always a shock because you never know what the strange object is going to turn out to be. Up it bursts; is it a psychosis, insanity—diagnosis please somebody!—genius, philosopher, poet, musician, composer? Then, while you try to survive *that,* whatever it is, up bursts your BODY shrieking for attention and complaining of neglect.

Your letter caused me—your fault!—to get out my paints and pour a lot of yellow and red over an unoffending piece of good white

[1] 'Estrangement', William Watson, 1858-1936.

paper. This masterpiece is called 'An Impression of Sunset'. It makes me angry whenever I catch sight of it. I suppose I shall have to let it dry before I can tear it up; tearing up *wet* paper is *so* unrewarding.

* * *

The Shah of Persia seems to have let off a land mine in the shape of Khomeini. I though that downy old bird would stick to his cosy nest in Paris but apparently even he has been blown out of Paris into Teheran by a sudden eruption of sincere Islamic belief.

I have been reading Kipling; an old friend and also a great friend to your Bion grandfather's profession—Indian Public Works (irrigation). I find depths in him I had forgotten (or never knew). These I have had brought to my notice by Birkenhead's very good biography. Mrs Bambridge[1] must have been as big a vandal as Lady Churchill was to Sutherland's portrait.[2] Disgraceful!

* * *

[1] Kipling's daughter.
[2] To these two might be added Lady Burton, wife of the explorer Richard Burton who translated *The Arabian Nights* and *The Perfumed Garden. see The Devil Drives*, Fawn M. Brodie, W. W. Norton & Co. Inc., 1967.

1976

Your beano with the patient who is alleged to have been negligently treated reminds me of one of my old chiefs—Bill Williams—who said, "The first thing you do before touching a fracture is be sure your malpractice insurance is in good shape; *then* have it X-rayed; set it; X-ray it again and damn the expense. Unfortunately you can only do the first thing in my job and the rest is in the lap of the gods. One of the first cases I had—of course it is when you are most vulnerable at the beginning of your career, and then when you are vulnerable because you are senile—was a paranoid girl who wanted to sue me. Luckily the malpractice people in England are very unflappable and unless you are patently guilty of being a nit-wit they stand by you. However, it is nasty while it lasts and heaven knows what a welfare state does for a doctor. Anyway an early inoculation stands you in good stead, unless of course the inoculation becomes inflamed.

* * *

We went out to dinner and had a very enjoyable and peculiar evening. Where, I wonder, outside a Jewish party, would time be taken up reading Keats's 'Ode to a Nightingale', two Shakespeare sonnets, two Milton sonnets; discussing the prospect of death; the preoccupation with the same; and the very noisy description of 'How I caught my husband' by the wife of an eminent cultural historian who has just completed (at age 92) the last, umpteenth volume of his history of cultural development? She was then so vulgarly and noisily offensive to Dr B. (who had been telling me about his medical care of and social friendship with Stravinsky) that he and his wife left the party in a rage.

At the end the hostess said how much she had missed the chance of speaking to me, though I was seated on her right hand through dinner! She was quite right of course—the racket was so great!

* * *

The path of true love is punctuated with divorce as well as marriage; the problem is, *when?* Before, after or during? It is a decision which is made by two people, both—oddly and painfully enough—in isolation. You always regret it, plus or minus: if it's a success, that it wasn't earlier; if it's a failure, ditto. And anyhow that it *might* have been better to do *the other thing* at a better time. As Sir Ronald Adam said to me about war: "No victory is so wonderful and complete, no disaster so disastrous as it looks". And he had reason to know, as he was the Adjutant General of the army. Whether you look at life through a microscope or a 200-inch telescope on Mount Palomar, it's much the same. Not very consoling perhaps, but—such is life.

We had a good trip to Topeka for our Friday, Saturday and half Sunday congress.[1] We both had doubts of the wisdom of it as I supposed there would be about 100 people and I was the last speaker on the programme, by which time I supposed everyone would have disappeared to their respective hutches, homes, warrens or whatever it was from which they originally had emerged. We waited in a hotel lounge specially set apart for us at the airport at Kansas City and eventually about six of us collected and off we went on our 90-odd mile ride to Topeka. Now— this was at Kansas. Kansas City? No. Kansas. Oh I see—this is in Kansas State. M'p'raps; p'raps not. Eventually the bus passed through, in darkness now, Kansas. Kansas what? Kansas, Missouri. Oh, I suppose Kansas City of course is in Kansas State—the capital? No! No! NO! The capital of Kansas State is Topeka. Ah, yes. Of course. Stupid of me. Big town? Oh no—twenty or thirty thousand. Ah—there's the Missouri! Not *the* Missouri? Yes, *the* Missouri. Shades of Shenandoah and echoes in school days of that most enchanting of songs—'Away, I'm bound to go 'cross the wide Missouri.' I had never believed that one day I would cross the wide Missouri. And no number of bridges and factories could ever obliterate that fascinating, to me, love song.

Next morning I discovered that the congress was international and there were 760 members. Things, I felt, were looking up although I thought that most of them would have disappeared before my last item on Sunday. They hadn't. And as I never read my papers but talk direct to the audience, I think they found it quite a relief. I talked too long—too much to say.[2] I enjoyed myself and the whole outfit stuck it out till I had finished. We both started home weary, but glad to have come.

* * *

[1] Conference on Borderline Personality Disorders. Conference papers published by International Universities Press Inc., 1977.

[2] His prepared paper was 'Emotional Turbulence'; his talk, 'On a Quotation from Freud'.

I am bound to say I loved my utterly brainless and sensuous spasm of Oxford before reality closed down on me and I found I had no brain available for exam passing. One never really recovers from saying goodbye to the University. Bittersweet it is, alas! Bittersweet, but one cannot grudge the price.

Don't have anything to do with people who misjudge your abilities. Don't *cause* them to under-rate you. But whatever anyone else thinks, don't let them fool you, plus or minus. And your secret knowledge of who you are is the most important opinion of all, and *that* you do not have to make public. If you meet the right person you do gradually, and secretly, get to know more who he or she is and, at the same time, do find out to your surprise something of who you are. You do not however need to verbalize it—unless of course you are a psycho-analyst, and even then you do not have to do it ALOUD. I love to hear and see murmurations of starlings in England. But murmurations of human beings, NO. Unlike starlings, they are so dull. I remember having a shot at a starling just outside my window at Queen's with a small finger catapult. I aimed—and hit—just below him. He was 'chuckling' as they do; and was so surprised he stopped at once, cocked his head on one side, and looked at where the pellet hit as much as to say, "What *was* that?" Then he went on chuckling and saying, "My—what a glorious day!" I love starlings so much they almost bring tears to my eyes.

* * *

'Soft as old Sorrow, Bright as old Renown'—that sums up England as far as I'm concerned. Or perhaps I ought to say, some tiny part of England like Tom Quad with Great Tom sounding the curfew at Oxford, or my room at Queen's late at night reading Manley Hopkins:

'Some candle clear burns somewhere I come by.
I muse at how its being puts . . .'[1]

But read it yourself. I read it one horrible, dark foggy evening, and although I didn't understand it, it hit me so hard I learned it by heart and have learned it over and over again. I have never ceased to admire him.

* * *

[1] 'The Candle Indoors'.

We used to sing, with much vim and not a glimmer of a sense of humour, 'It is high time to awake, to awake out of sleep! For now is our salvation nearer than when we believ-ed.' Now I see that it was a superb anthem for the last Sunday of term. Life is funny—if only we could see the joke—which we never do. You remember G. K. Chesterton saying how right the printers were when they printed his most solemn passage about the 'cosmic' as 'comic'?

* * *

How difficult life is! Should I call you "darling" or "dear" or, or what? My mother used to call me "darling" till I became an officer with a DSO. Then she dropped it because her darling had disappeared in a sort of bog of GLORY.

* * *

Your story of the little owl reminded me of when I was staying at Burford watching a Lilford owl standing, intently gazing at a small haystack. I threw a pebble into the straw near him to see what he would do. He did not fly away, he did *not* leap on the pebble. He just turned his head slowly round and stared into my eyes. He looked daggers (perhaps I should say 'claws') at me as if to say, "You must be a bloody fool if you think I am such a bloody fool!" Then when—not before—he had decided "It's not funny!" he flew off. No wonder we think owls are wise.

* * *

Today the sun has come out for the first time since it started to rain three days ago. They say it's the first tropical storm they have had in L.A. since 1934. Well, we wanted rain. "Lord, Lord! We have prayed for rain but this is just fair rideecilous!" as the parson is said to have petitioned the Almighty in his church.

* * *

You must be going through that ghastly post-Varsity stage during which most people discover that they have lost all their chances—marriage, jobs, First Class Honours, and the rest. In another twenty years (30? 40? 50? 60?) you discover that you might have been unlucky and been 'successful'. Not that that is much consolation while you are licking your wounds; the wounds are too sore.

* * *

Many thanks for your Seurat[1]—I don't think I have seen it. I imagine he was trying to create the impression of brilliant sunlight though it does look rather like mist—so does bright sunlight of course; it is not helped by the fact that the artist has to use an opaque medium like oil colours. (As I find if I try to paint here.)

[1] 'Gravelines', in the Courtauld Collection, London.

1977

I keep wanting to buy some ludicrously expensive, new and improved household gadget, but I am at last beginning to be slightly sales-resistant though I still fall for books forgetting that you can't wear them or eat them and they take a long time to read.

Many people mistake the practice of psycho-analysis for an adequate substitute for real life. I don't know what 'real life' is, but I am jolly sure that psycho-analysis is no good unless it resembles it. 'A prelude to—*not* a substitute for—' I try to tell them. 'A substitute is a substitute is a substitute', as Gertrude Stein might have said.

* * *

I am glad your visit to France was rewarding even as a rest for your mind and a chance for an airing of your bodily capacities. I hope your muscles have recovered and that you are not now experiencing too violent a battering of your mental capacity. The great thing about having such experiences is that in the course of balancing one thing against another you *also* get a clue to *who* you are. And more still, you become YOU. 'I have six honest serving men' says Kipling in *Just So Stories.* A great and good man despite his unfortunate obsession with Stalky and Co.—the British Army which is so much more stupid than he allowed himself to realize. But all institutions are stupid and try to crush the individuals inside them. If not by blame, then praise. 'Treat both those imposters alike'—as Kipling again says.

At present I am suffering a momentary dose of 'success' which I try to do without being caught by surprise when the next bash comes; or having my pleasant interlude eroded by preoccupations with the next unknown horrors!

Mummy is overworking but don't tell her I said so. These Mothers get awfully shirty if fussed over.

1978

It's a rum life when one cannot have a leisurely and pleasing opportunity even of writing to one's daughter who in any case is carried at enormous speed into the category of 'old friend'—if one is lucky. At one moment a baby daughter and at the next, so it seems, a young woman with a life and thoughts and ideas of her own. 'Eheu fugaces, Postume, Postume . . .' Horace knew a thing or two.[1] I sometimes feel that if I am lucky I can only boast of knowing one thing and not much of that. Still, psycho-analysis, in so far as I know it, is not bad—there might be worse professions. Sometimes I feel that it is only 'by accident' that I am so well off and indeed it is only thanks to the accidents that I am as well off as I am.

*   *   *

It is always hard to achieve a success so one is sometimes liable to snatch at the first that offers and regret it, or be choosey and turn it down (and regret that!). So, sometimes it is nice to feel that one appears to have got it *right*. Especially as one never has settled things 'once for all'. It opens up a new and greater crop of problems whenever you settle one. Still—it can be fun.

Envy and rivalry and hate are so prevalent that they seem to be the spiritual nutrition on which we have to live.

*   *   *

When you muse about, and mourn your multitudinous failings—take courage. You are not the only one. Luckily for me I happened on a very efficient and charming girl (your Mother) or else I too would be mouldering 'sous la terre' of Iver Heath. Or—it is frightening to realize it—in a job in the Veterans Administration which was offered me after the last war. Incidentally I can't help wondering how it doesn't seem to occur to anyone that the reason why we are so poor is that it is very expensive to fight *two* wars and to be the only nation that was in both of them from start to finish and did *not* lose either of them.

*   *   *

[1] Horace, Ode XIV. 'Alas, Postumus, the fleeting years are slipping by.'

I hope soon to be able to send you some material—research into cot deaths here. The findings are I think much the same as those in England—an allergy, possibly connected with the milk on which the baby is fed.

If you care to develop, or keep it under your hat for future use, I send you a hunch of my own. (Hunch=untested, unsupported day-dream of psycho-analyst which may or may not be worth investigating. *Not* even a theory.)

A sub-sensible (i.e. available to the senses) disturbance of food functioning, e.g. breast, *might*, if allowed to develop to point where it became diagnosible as 'diabetes', exist in a primitive, rudimentary, embryonic or embryo-carrying mother, and disturb the mother's productions, and the products, ultimately, of the infant.

1. Examples of mother's products: babies, faeces, urine, sweat, milk.

2. Necessary pathological biochemical investigations: urine, for sugar—almost certainly done anyhow; sweat, for sugar; faeces, for sugar. This would be difficult to do because necessary to find reagents of adequate degree of sensitivity. When I asked Himsworth, the then head of the Medical Research Council, if a patient he had referred to me had had her sweat tested for sugar when in coma (she was a diabetic), he—though then also the leading expert—was staggered and confessed "no". He also said he knew of no apparatus for testing. Professor Rosenheim was equally or more hostile to investigation—too superior to a 'bloody psycho-analyst' probably.

3. If the mother is excreting, in any form and by any channel—alimentary, genital or even respiratory—*pre cursors* of sugar or milk, the infant might then be 'allergic' after birth to the mother's sweat or milk.

Just a plausible (too plausible?) hunch. It may even bear on mysteries like eclampsia, psychoses of pregnancy etc. Key problems—cromaffin tissue, para sympathetic and sympathetic nervous systems, and subthalamic regions generally.

Don't lose your compassion for the strikers or your realization that a victory for dictatorship by anybody is a disaster even if democracy seems to be little good.

*　　*　　*

I am drawing near to a lunch on Saturday next in my honour. That will I think be the last of these flattering but onerous occasions.[1] Though these intentions are well meant (tarantara![2]) they are *not* calculated to cheer yours truly, WRB.

Thank you very much for sending off the books from Blackwells. It is always exciting to have new books although one *knows* that one has no space for them or time to read them. It is an addiction; it looks respectable but is not.

I have been reading the Mahabarata and wondering why it is familiar. Then it dawned on me it must be because it was the sort of tale my old Ayah must have told me—on and on and on, incredible, incomprehensible, a survival of Sanskrit stories which must be about the oldest in the world. *Then* I came across a bit which is indistinguishable from a part of Kung Fu—isn't that incredible?—another ancient literature, the Chinese civilization. I am just beginning to think I ought to go to Oxford and get educated. And India; and Peking. In short—again. A bit late, as I should also include Rome and Latin. Eheu fugaces!

[1] His eightieth birthday.
[2] *The Pirates of Penzance*, Gilbert and Sullivan.

1979

Do not get misled by gross statements of what 'Ch'i' means—there is no simple translation of it—not even from Chinese to Chinese. Western articulate speech probably comes nearer, as far as I can see it, in Schopenhauer's 'drive' or 'energy', or Alf Arabi's 'existence'.

I, to descend from the famous to the nonentity, make a distinction between 'existence', to be or not to be (Shakespeare as usual says it better than anyone has been able to say it) and 'essence', the whatever-it-is that makes existence worth existing. That is what no one can tell you, and what every philosopher, painter, musician, artist, poet and mere person has to find out for him or her self. I'll write a book about it one day p'raps, p'raps not. That's what your patients, however ill, well, wealthy, poor, stupid, clever, have to find out. They can't be shown, but you may give them a chance to see or find out.

* * *

A wonderful, bright and sunny morning—wind and rain both stopped, just for the day perhaps but a welcome rest—'Full many a glorious morning have I seen—'[1] as the sonnet has it. Do you read them? They are short and the meaning, as with everything W.S. says, unfolds meaning after meaning through one's life. Indeed that is the wonderful thing about medicine and I wish I had realized it when I had the luck to be studying at UCH. But, as at Oxford, one does not, always being preoccupied with some infernal anxiety about 'qualification' or 'Finals' or how to earn a living or some other worry to fuss about. Including of course, 'she loves me—she loves me not—' and 'Do I love her—do I *not*', like the child's game with plucking petals from a flower (or leaves from a pineapple—the Queen's College version of the sweepstake when I was up).

Talking of Shakespeare, I have recently decided, after a long sojourn in the gloomy realms of ghastly good taste in which Gilbert and Sullivan are really not worthy of serious consideration, that in fact they are packed with great sense as well as being witty and amusing.

I continue after the interruption—your phone call!—which was a very pleasant surprise. It makes a wonderful difference that one can

[1] Sonnet 33.

have these artificial aids to communication; one thinks the Dark Ages (new style) have their compensations.

* * *

I wish we could all meet, but this is a peculiarity of Old Age Greed!

ENVOI[1]

One day in April 1951, soon after Wilfred and I had announced our engagement, I was going up in the lift to my office at the Tavistock Institute in the company of John Harvard Watts, who said, 'I hear you are going to nurture genius'. This was a surprising and somewhat intimidating challenge; it conjured up images of an eccentric; a recuse; an absent-minded intellectual with a disregard for his personal appearance, a lack of interest in food, hollow-cheeked, of fragile health. But none of these seemed to fit this man with whom I wanted to spend the rest of my life. *He* was shy, modest, affectionate, witty and of marked robust health; a lover of good food, wine and the best cigars. So I felt confident in accepting John's remark as friendly flattery.

But he was right. I had not then met the iron man who existed within the benevolent one. His determination not to be moulded into a shape congenial to others, his courage in forging ahead with work he *felt* was on the right track although he could present no evidence to prove his feelings, his refusal to be or do anything untrue to himself—these, combined with a penetrating insight into the human mind and the human condition, produced an extraordinary person. And because the iron never entered his soul he remained highly sensitive and receptive to any thoughts or ideas floating around looking for a mind to lodge in.

His view of himself, however, was so different from that held by those of us who admired and loved him that it was difficult to recognize any relationship. He complained again and again, when we were talking together, of his ignorance and what he called his 'gutlessness'; he totally rejected descriptions of himself as 'outstanding' or 'famous'. He would quote, 'There are no fields of amaranth this side of the grave. There are no voices that are not soon mute however tuneful. There is no name with whatever emphasis of passionate love repeated of which the echo is not faint at last.' 'You're a

[1] **Delivered to the British Psycho-Analytical Society on 20, February 1980 and published in the International Review of Psycho-Analysis, 1981. Reproduced here by kind permission of the Editor.**

pessimist' I would say, trying not to weep. 'No', he would reply, 'just a realist.'

It takes courage to be a realist and true courage goes hand in hand with fear. He *was* afraid—as a small boy separated from his parents, at school in a strange country; as a tank commander in the First World War, going into battle knowing that the chance of survival after the third attack was nil; as a psycho-analyst facing the terrors of the unknown; even as a lecturer addressing an audience without the life-belt of a handful of printed pages. I know that this took great courage. He would often say to me, with a look of alarm, just before 'going on stage' as it were, 'But I've nothing to say', or, 'Whatever am I going to say to them?' He did not in fact know beforehand what he was going to say. What we heard was freshly minted, even new to *him*; there would appear a phrase, a sentence I had not heard him use before—a bright flash of insight, leaving an afterglow in the mind's eye.

Poetry was of central importance to him all his life. He often spoke of the unforgettable impact that certain poets had on him during his school days—Milton, Virgil, Shakespeare, Keats, Shelley—it says much for his school that he was not forced into hating the poets before he had had time to love them.

All beautiful things moved him to tears—whether it was poetry, prose, music, painting, sculpture, or the Norfolk landscape, its sea birds and its skylarks. In a letter written to me a few days after we first met he said, 'It is a marvellous moonlit night with the wind sighing gently in the pine trees. There is a line of Flecker's which goes, "For pines are gossip pines the wide world through". It has always stuck in my mind since I first came across it when I was at Oxford. Arthur Bryant and I used to learn quite a lot of verse when I was up. But I think I learnt most during the first war. My biggest feat was in 1918 when our battalion had no tanks left, and I and a dozen of my men had to fill a gap in the line with our machine guns. Our last night before relief I was with a colonel of the Royal Scots and it became clear as we were talking that a German night attack was starting. As everything that could be done had been done he said, "Let's talk about something decent". So we talked about the Roger de Coverly essays while the Germans shelled to bits our water-logged line of shell holes and earthworks. The colonel got killed a little later and I, still having nothing to do, learned L'Allegro and Il Penseroso from a Golden Treasury I had with me.'

It is not surprising then, that he had hoped to compile an anthology of poetry; and since psycho-analysis was fundamental to his thinking, the collection was to be for psycho-analysts. Not, he said, for anyone who is merely *called* a psycho-analyst, not the label of certification, but the 'real thing'. The pieces were to be selected, not for the practice of psycho-analytic virtuosity in giving so-called 'psycho-analytic' interpretations, but because a psycho-analytically expanded capacity would fit the reader to have a new experience, however familiar he might think he was with previous experience of the words.

Unfortunately the anthology will have to join the long list of his projected but unwritten works, but I would like to read to you part of what he wrote as an introduction.

It is easy in this age of the plague—not of poverty and hunger, but of plenty, surfeit and gluttony—to lose our capacity for awe. It is as well to be reminded by the poet Herman Melville that there are many ways of reading books, but very few of reading them properly—that is, with awe. How much the more is it true of reading people.

Someone asked, 'Why climb mountains?' 'Because they are there' was the reply. I would add that there are some who would prefer to postpone the exercise till their rugosities, heights, depths and declivities have been worn to a uniform flatness. The Grand Canyon will be tamed; Everest, Kanchenjunga neon-lit; the pass of Glencoe deserted by its ghosts; Nanda Devi no longer the home of the Seven Rishis; the Master of Stair a phantom without bones. William Blake, in Gnomic Verses said, 'Great things are done when men and mountains meet; This is not done by jostling in the street'.

I resort to the poets because they seem to me to say something in a way which is beyond my powers and yet to be in a way which I myself would choose *if* I had the capacity. The unconscious—for want of a better word—seems to me to show the way 'down to descend', its realms have an awe-inspiring quality.

One of Wilfred's two copies of Robert Bridges' *Spirit of Man* shows signs of many years handling and reading; some of the poems are marked with a pencil line in the margin; some of the marks are of double or treble thickness showing increasing degrees of enthusiasm. On the blank pages he wrote some poems and quotations of his own choice, among them a poem by Flecker, 'To a Poet a Thousand Years Hence'.

At the time of Wilfred's death Julian, discovering the truth of Blake's words, 'meeting mountains', was trekking round Annapurna. He would like to add this poem to those we read at the cremation.

I who am dead a thousand years
And wrote this sweet archaic song
Send you my words for messengers
The way I shall not pass along.

I care not if you bridge the seas
Or ride secure the cruel sky
Or build consummate palaces
Of metal or of masonry.

But have you wine and music still,
And statues and a bright-eyed love,
And foolish thoughts of good or ill,
And prayers to them who sit above?

How shall we conquer? Like a wind
That falls at eve our fancies blow,
And old Maeonides the blind
Said it three thousand years ago.

O friend unseen, unborn, unknown,
Student of our sweet English tongue,
Read out my words at night alone,
I was a poet, I was young.

Since I can never see your face
And never shake you by the hand,
I send my soul through time and space
To greet you. You will understand.

He died as he had lived—with courage. He accepted the end of his life philosophically, adhering to his belief in the advice, 'Do not strive officiously to keep alive.' On 14 November we stood in Happisburgh churchyard on the cliffs high above the North Sea. Here, in his 'beloved Norfolk' of bracing winds, wide skies, bright light, dear to him since boyhood, the ashes were buried; here he was always happy.

He would often quote this poem of George Herbert's on waking to a morning of sunlight—hastening to add that many thought it poor verse, but he found it beautiful.

ENVOI

Virtue

Sweet day, so cool, so calm, so bright!
The bridal of the earth and sky—
The dew shall weep thy fall tonight;
For thou must die.

Sweet rose, whose hue angry and brave
Bids the rash gazer wipe his eye,
Thy root is ever in its grave,
And thou must die.

Sweet spring, full of sweet days and roses,
A box where sweets compacted lie,
My music shows ye have your closes,
And all must die.

Only a sweet and virtuous soul,
Like season'd timber, never gives;
But though the whole world turn to coal,
Then chiefly lives.

My grand-daughter, aged seven, put into words what so many of us felt after Wilfred's death—'I didn't realize I knew Grandpa so well.' His love, wisdom, affectionate humour, sympathetic concern permeated our lives. I believe we shall continue to feel, sometimes with surprise, that we didn't realize we knew him so well.

FRANCESCA BION

For Product Safety Concerns and Information please contact our EU representative GPSR@taylorandfrancis.com Taylor & Francis Verlag GmbH, Kaufingerstraße 24, 80331 München, Germany

Batch number: 10725893

Printed by Printforce, the Netherlands